Quality Project

Josh K. Early

Abstract

Overweight and obesity are a constant problem among patients seen at the project site. There was no guideline to provide a framework to manage overweight and obese patients at the project site. The purpose of this quantitative quasi-experimental quality improvement project was to determine if the implementation of the American Heart Association, American College of Cardiology, and The Obesity Society (AHA/ACC/TOS) *Guidelines for the Management of Overweight and Obesity in Adults* would impact weight, body mass index (BMI), and obesity risk knowledge among adults with BMI greater than 25 kg/m^2. The project was completed over four weeks in a primary care clinic in central California. Imogene King's theory of goal attainment and Hochbaum and Rosenstock's health belief model were the theoretical frameworks used for the project. The Agency for Healthcare Research and Quality's Tool 2 chart audit form and Obesity Risk Knowledge-10 were used to collect data among the sample of 28 patients. A paired *t*-test revealed a clinical and statistically significant change in patient weight (t (27) = 4.01, p=.000); BMI (t(27)=3.44, p=.002); and obesity risk knowledge score (t(21)= -26.95, p=.000). Therefore, implementing the AHA/ACC/TOS *Guidelines for the Management of Overweight and Obesity in Adults* may improve weight, BMI, and knowledge in this population and setting. Recommendations include sustaining the project and dissemination of the results.

Keywords: American Heart Association, American College of Cardiology, The Obesity Society, Agency for Healthcare Research and Quality Tool 2 chart audit form, obesity risk knowledge, overweight, obesity, primary care, King's theory of goal attainment, health belief model.

Table of Contents

List of Tables

List of Figures

Chapter 1: Introduction

Overweight and obesity are among the greatest health issues in the United States (Hales et al., 2020). Adult obesity in the United States (U.S.) is an ongoing health problem for greater than 70% of the population (Hales et al., 2020). According to Hales et al. (2020), 31% and 43& of adults are overweight and obese respectively in U.S. Obesity and overweight contribute to a significant risk for type 2 diabetes mellitus (T2DM), cardiovascular disease (CVD), hypertension, and stroke, and certain forms of cancer (Ryu et al., 2019). The health consequences range from increased risk of premature death to severe chronic conditions that reduce an individual's overall quality of life. Given the current weight management background and rising overweight and obesity levels, research suggested that studies had not yet presented a sustainable weight management program. This quantitative direct practice improvement project was supported by established evidence that defined the relationship between offering weight management opportunities using clinical guidelines in the primary care setting versus current practice with outcome data.

The management of overweight and obesity often was addressed during office visits at the primary care project site; however, patients were given little ongoing weight management and instructed to lose weight without detailed information or guidance on what intervention to take (Hayes, 2019). Advanced practice nurses (APNs) are uniquely positioned to identify those at risk for overweight and obesity, assess and screen for complications, and educate and treat patients as recommended by overweight and obesity clinical guidelines (Hayes, 2019; Puente & Martinez-Marcos, 2018). The APNs use evidenced-based practice guidelines in all aspects of nursing care to be an integral part of clinical practice to optimize patient outcomes, improve quality of care, and contain costs. (Bourgault, 2018; Wilkerson et al., 2018). However, research suggested that APNs commonly underutilized overweight and obesity management guidelines and did not have adequate knowledge to treat overweight and obese patients (Hayes, 2019). Since APNs increasingly served as the primary source of care for patients, the APNs should value the need to address and treat the growing problem of obesity in the U.S. to improve patient outcomes related to weight loss and obesity risk knowledge. In 2018, The Obesity Society (TOS) first published a position statement on obesity as a chronic disease that should be managed like other chronic diseases (Jastreboff et al., 2019). According to Bray et al. (2017), only recently has obesity become a popular topic for the medical community. Obesity had grown into a major healthcare concern in the U.S.

This project evaluated whether the implementation of the American Heart Association (AHA), American College of Cardiology (ACC), and The Obesity Society (TOS) guidelines would positively impact patient outcomes for overweight and obese patients in the primary care setting. The AHA, ACC, and TOS guidelines were published in 2014 to provide the best evidence to assist primary care providers (PCPs) in making the best clinical decisions for overweight and obese patients (Jensen et al., 2014). It was proposed that the utilization of AHA, ACC, and TOS guidelines for weight management facilitated in the primary care setting would benefit the patient population. This direct practice improvement project utilized the AHA, ACC, and TOS guidelines for a weight management program that offered dietary advice and exercised encouragement to patients at the project site to help close this gap. The TOS suggested that considering obesity a disease is likely to have more positive outcomes than negative consequences and to benefit the greater good by providing resources for prevention and treatment (Jastreboff et al., 2019). Obesity as a chronic disease will be encouraged by caring healthcare professionals to view treating the obese patient as a disease like other chronic diseases (Sharma & Campbell-Scherer, 2017). The new guidelines' overarching message by TOS was that no single eating pattern was best for overweight or obese patients (Jastreboff et al., 2019). The key to achieving optimal health and nutrition for weight loss was individualization focusing on a low-calorie diet of patient choice (Jastreboff et al., 2019).

Chapter 1 introduces this direct practice improvement (DPI) project. It includes discussing the project's background, purpose, problem statement, clinical questions, and how it advances scientific knowledge. The project's significance, the rationale for the methodology, nature of the research design, definition of terms, assumptions, limitations, delimitations, and the project's summary and organization are also discussed in this chapter.

Background of the Project

Worldwide, adult obesity had tripled over the last 40 years, rising from 205 million in 1975 to 641 million in 2016 (Centers for Disease Control and Prevention [CDC], 2017). Overweight and obesity rates had reached 35% in 7 states, 30% in 29 states, and 25% in 48 states (CDC, 2018). According to World Health Organization (WHO, 2018), health organizations have recognized overweight and obesity as a threat to the nation's well-being. The medical costs for obese patients are between 36-150% higher than non-obesity patients (Public Health, 2018). Using data from 2006-2013, the medical costs of obese adults in 2013 dollars is $3429 higher than non-obese individuals (Biener et al., 2017). Obesity equates to about $150 billion spent in healthcare annually (Segal et al., 2017). Indirect costs are difficult to ascertain but include absenteeism, increased transportation costs related to fuel, and health insurance costs totaling $988.8 billion (Segal et al., 2017). The estimated indirect and direct costs for individuals with obesity were $1.42 trillion in 2014 (Segal et al., 2017).

Obesity is considered a chronic disease (Hale & Mangoo, 2021; Hayes et al., 2017). While the TOS declared obesity as a disease in 2008, the American Medical Association (AMA) did not follow suit until 2013; the AMA categorized obesity as a complex, chronic disease requiring medical intervention (Fitzpatrick & Steven, 2017). In addition to chronic diseases, obesity frequently was accompanied by gallbladder disease, breast cancer, endometrial cancer, colon cancer, and osteoarthritis (Dewhurst et al., 2017). There has been a 28.9% increase in death and disability related to obesity between 1990 and 2016 (Institute for Health Metrics and Evaluation [IHME], 2018). It was estimated that at least 2.8 million people might die each year worldwide from being obese (Malambo et al., 2017).

Over the past decades, management of overweight and obesity in the primary care setting utilizing evidence-based guidelines had been lacking (Fitzpatrick & Steven, 2017; Hayes, 2019). Management of overweight and obese adults involved clinical guidelines based on evidence-based practice to guide PCPs to improve patients' health outcomes (Jensen et al., 2014). Evidence illustrates that despite the recommendation to screen adults for obesity and overweight, the number of individuals diagnosed is low (Hayes, 2019). Fitzpatrick and Steven (2017) state most electronic health records calculate the body mass index (BMI) for the provider; however, the provider must add the diagnosis to the problem list. The documentation of overweight and obesity in the problem list occurs in less than 30% of patients leading to a gap in current practice. The patients with a diagnosis were more likely to receive weight-loss counseling or treatment. Increasing the patients' diagnosis for overweight and obesity is the foundation to change the trajectory of the disease of obesity and overweight. This project focused on the AHA, ACC, and TOS guidelines for managing overweight and obese adults in the primary care setting. Reis et al. (2018) examined the quality of clinical guidelines for managing overweight and obese adults using the appraisal of guidelines for research and evaluation (AGREE). The following criteria were included: (1) clinical guidelines for overweight and obesity, (2) treatment recommendations for adults, and (3) involvement of a government agency and state-level societies of health professionals (Reis et al., 2018; Tchang et al., 2021).

Problem Statement

It was not known if or to what degree the implementation of the American Heart Association, American College of Cardiology, and The Obesity Society (AHA/ACC/TOS) *Guidelines for the Management of Overweight and Obesity in Adults* would impact weight, body mass index (BMI), and obesity risk knowledge among adults with BMI greater than 25 kg/m2. The obstacle at the project site was the lack of clinical guidelines or protocol for APNs to assess and manage the overweight and obese patient. Thus, the practice site did not offer patients a designated evidence-based intervention focused on weight management because APNs did not acknowledge obesity as a chronic disease. The management of overweight and obesity is never discussed or included in a problem list during an office visit at the project site. The patients usually were verbally informed to watch their diet regardless of their class of BMI. The recording and measurement of weight by ancillary staff and verbal instruction to watch their diet and exercise formed a part of the routine office visits when APNs encounter overweight or obese patients.

The population selected for this project was adults with BMI greater than 25 kg/m^2. The rationale for opting for the age group was that the intervention was specifically developed for adults in a primary care setting. The majorities of overweight and obese patients who visit the project site are independent and usually present to the clinic alone. The participants under age 18 will require parents or guidance permission to participate in the project.

Despite numerous resources such as clinical practice guidelines, algorithms, and treatment models, there is a gap in APNs' approach to treating overweight and obesity at the project site. While literature indicated that the clinical guidelines such as AHA, ACC, and TOS were evidence-based used to assess for overweight and obesity, it was not known at the primary care project site located in central California to what degree the AHA, ACC, and TOS guidelines would help to improve patient outcomes (Hayes et al., 2017).

The primary care project site in central California has observed an increase in overweight and obese patients in the last three years. The highest numbers of patients seen at the project site are obese Hispanics. The central region of California is one of the nation's leading agricultural areas. Central California was also one of the poorest regions, where the highest populations in central California are Hispanic, and overweight and obesity were prevalent (Elflein, 2020). Hispanics also had a significantly higher prevalence of obesity than non-Hispanic whites and non-Hispanic blacks (CDC, 2017). Therefore, there was a need for an intervention to improve overweight and obese issues faced by individuals in the central California primary project site. Efforts to bring a degree of attention to utilizing evidence-based clinical guidelines with AHA, ACC, and TOS to identify and manage overweight and obese patients have proven unsuccessful. This project contributed to identifying overweight, obesity, and patients at risk of obesity-related complications by introducing the AHA, ACC, and TOS guidelines to the project site. By implementing the AHA, ACC, TOS guidelines, measurable interventions were applied to the current practice. The AHA, ACC, and TOS guidelines have been shown by evidence to improve weight loss outcomes and increase awareness of obesity-related complications (Fitzpatrick & Steven, 2017).

Research has recently begun to explore the feasibility of providing weight-loss counseling to overweight and obese patients as part of their routine care in the primary care office (Berger et al., 2019; McVay et al., 2019; Nair & Hart, 2018; Torre et al., 2018). Another study explored how weight counseling provision using clinical guidelines contributed to increasing knowledge and improved obesity treatment (Osmundsen et al., 2019). Little was known about changes in diet or physical activity when counseling was provided by PCPs. Using a longitudinal randomized controlled trial, Halbert et al. (2017) examined the changes in eating behaviors and physical activity. The authors predicted weight loss outcomes among 282 obese adults who participated in a two-year behavioral weight loss intervention. Halbert et al. (2017) concluded that interventions with PCPs resulted in clinically meaningful weight loss in some patients, with corresponding improvements in low-calorie diet and energy expenditure. Based on this study's information, intervention from the PCPs utilizing evidence-based clinical guidelines could contribute to solving the problem of weight management at the project site.

This direct practice improvement project aimed to solve the project's site practice problem by proposing evidence-based guidelines for weight management that would positively impact weight reduction by introducing the AHA, ACC, and TOS guidelines. This project offered the opportunity for APNs to provide a practice improvement that produced data to establish weight management at the project site, closing a practice gap, and meeting quality measures. The evidence-based AHA, ACC, and TOS guidelines included a low-calorie diet and exercise and had improved patient outcomes (Al-Nimr et al., 2020; Jensen et al., 2014; Turner et al., 2018). Despite evidence demonstrating weight loss using evidence-based clinical guidelines efficacy, providers listed lack of awareness as the most common reason for not treating overweight and obesity (Fruh et al., 2019; Granara & Laurent, 2017). Patients with comorbidities are most likely to be offered weight-loss-loss intervention, indicating a late intervention or a missed opportunity to prevent co-morbidity by intervening earlier in the disease process (Granara & Laurent, 2017). Implementing the AHA/ACC/TOS guidelines by APNs may help close the awareness and knowledge gap to identify and treat overweight and obese patients and prevent other chronic diseases.

Purpose of the Project

The purpose of this quantitative quasi-experimental quality improvement project was to determine if the implementation of the American Heart Association, American College of Cardiology, and The Obesity Society (AHA/ACC/TOS) *Guidelines for the Management of Overweight and Obesity in Adults* would impact weight, body mass index (BMI), and obesity risk knowledge among adults with BMI greater than 25 kg/m^2. The project was completed over four weeks in a primary care clinic in central California. The

AHA, ACC, TOS guidelines (independent variable) are step-by-step instructions for managing overweight and obesity in primary care settings (Jensen et al., 2014). The AHA, ACC, TOS guidelines have been proven reliable for managing overweight and obesity in the primary care setting (Bays et al., 2019; Mechanick et al., 2017; Reis et al., 2018). The dependent variables of change in weight, BMI, and obesity risk knowledge were measured pre-intervention and post-intervention to determine the impact of the guidelines for managing overweight and obesity at the project site.

The project aim was to determine if the implementation of AHA, ACC, and TOS guidelines by APNs showed a reduction in weight and BMI after a four-week intervention. The project also explored whether there was a change in obesity risk knowledge among those with BMI greater than 30 kg/m2 who completed the intervention based on AHA, ACC, and TOS guidelines. The AHA, ACC, and TOS guidelines were used to identify and select participants at risk for obesity-related diseases based on the BMI. According to the 2014 guidelines and based on substantial evidence, even a modest, sustained weight loss of 3% to 5% will result in clinically meaningful health benefits for a patient with obesity risk factors (T2DM, CVD, and cancers).

Clinical Question

Preventing any disease, including overweight and obesity, is substantially less costly than disease treatment (CDC, 2017). Prevention of obesity in adults can be achieved through healthy lifestyle modifications, including a low–calorie diet and physical activity (Heymsfield et al., 2018). The intervention to improve the public health crisis of overweight and obesity requires evidence-based clinical guidelines (Wilkerson et al., 2018). Early recognition and treatment of overweight and obesity is the first step in prevention and treatment (Hayes, 2019; Winik & Bonham, 2018). Based on the gaps of evidence stated in the AHA, ACC, TOS guidelines for the management of overweight and obese adults, research is needed to understand better and improve the efficiency of lifestyle interventions in primary care settings. The project focused on introducing the AHA, ACC, and TOS guidelines to improve weight loss outcomes (decrease weight and BMI) and increased obesity risk knowledge at the project site. The AHA, ACC, and TOS guidelines were published in 2014 for PCPs for managing overweight and obese patients in a primary care setting (Jensen et al., 2014). Therefore, it is anticipated that this project of the 4-week intervention with the AHA, AHA, TOS guidelines as a reference would produce a reduction in weight, BMI, and increased obesity risk knowledge at the project site. The project answered the clinical question: To what degree would the implementation of the American Heart Association, American College of Cardiology, and The Obesity Society (AHA/ACC/TOS) *Guidelines for the Management of Overweight and Obesity in Adults* would impact weight, body mass index (BMI), and obesity risk knowledge among adults with BMI greater than 25 kg/m^2 in a primary care clinic in central California?

Advancing Scientific Knowledge

Obesity is considered a chronic disease (Hayes et al., 2017). Overweight and obesity persist for multiple reasons; it is not simply an issue of poor self-control concerning foods or a lack of motivation to move (Hayes et al., 2017). There are specific biochemical adaptations that characterize obesity as a chronic disease (Institute of Health Metrics and Evaluation, 2018). One contributing factor stands out: during annual well-visits, less than 50% of obese adults reported that their primary care physician addressed weight management (Hayes, 2019). Even though clinical practice guidelines are available, the under-treatment of overweight and obesity in primary care persists (Hayes, 2019; Heymsfield et al., 2018).

Evidence-based clinical guidelines are comprehensive lifestyle interventions used to address overweight and obesity management disparities in adult populations. AHA, ACC, and TOS guidelines were developed based on high-quality randomized trials, meta-analyses, and observational studies to identify, prevent, and treat overweight and obesity in a primary care setting (Jensen et al., 2014). The AHA, ACC, and TOS guidelines were used as a reference to assess weight, BMI, and obesity risk knowledge and determine if any changes between pre-and post-intervention. According to Reis et al. (2018), there was a lack of information about overweight and obesity lifestyle interventions for PCPs incorporating the AHA, ACC, and TOS guidelines. Jensen et al. (2014) recognized that research was needed to improve overweight and obesity in a primary care setting. Evidence has shown that management of obesity using evidence-based clinical guidelines improved the chronic diseases associated with obesity. Still, the PCPs, including the APNs in primary care settings, lack clinical guidelines while treating overweight and obesity (Jensen et al., 2014).

This project evaluated overweight and obese participants' clinical outcomes and identified those who achieved the recommended 3-5% weight loss according to the AHA, ACC, and TOS guidelines. According to Jensen et al. (2014), further research was needed to understand the treatment of overweight and obesity in a primary care setting and improve the efficiency of lifestyle interventions (low-calorie and increase physical activity). Disser (2019) examined the overweight and obesity treatment guidelines in a retrospective analysis. There was a statistically significant improvement in weight management documentation and anthropometric values after training sessions but limited intervention improvement. Reis et al. (2018) found that despite obesity clinical guidelines to promote overweight and obesity treatment, there was no statistically significant change in anthropometric markers' treatment or improvement. Overweight and obesity guidelines are available for review, complete with the chief recommendation to assess and treat adults as part of routine screening and wellness visits. Yet, PCPs have not followed through consistently (Hayes, 2019). Previous research revealed that PCPs, including APNs, could effectively manage overweight and obesity in the primary care setting (Heymsfield et al., 2018).

There are several evidence-based clinical guidelines for managing overweight and obesity for PCPs in primary care settings; many of these guidelines are still not known to the PCPs at the project site. Therefore, a gap in practice could be filled by implementing evidence-based clinical guidelines in primary care settings (Hayes, 2019). This project was focused on the AHA, ACC, and TOS guidelines. The utilization of AHA, ACC, and TOS guidelines at the project site by APNs will help the project manager evaluate overweight and obese participants' clinical outcomes and identified those who achieved the recommended 3-5% weight loss according to the guidelines. Implementing the evidence-based AHA, ACC, and TOS guidelines is the key to address, treat, and prevent overweight and obesity in adults in a primary care setting (Jensen et al., 2014). Intervention is critical to improving our nation's health and decreasing associated healthcare costs of a preventable chronic health condition associated with obesity. Therefore, it is anticipated that this project of the 4-week intervention that used AHA,

ACC, and TOS guidelines recommendations as a reference will provide insights related to weight-loss outcome and knowledge of obesity-related risk among overweight and obese adults at the project site.

This project was grounded in two theoretical underpinnings. The first foundation was based on Imogene King's theory of goal attainment (TGA). King developed the TGA in the early 1960s to describe an interpersonal relationship a patient developed to manage life goals (King, 1992). The assumption of TGA is that a nurse and client communicate information, set goals mutually, and act to attain the goals. The model has three interacting systems: personal, interpersonal, and social. Each of these systems has its own set of concepts. The personal system concepts are perception, self, growth and development, body image, space, and time. The concepts for the interpersonal system are interaction, communication, transaction, role, and stress. The concepts for the social system are the organization, authority, power, status, and decision-making. TGA was derived from the relationships in the theory of interacting systems. The scholarly project examined specific aspects of the interaction between APNs and patients, independent of AHA/ACC/TOS guidelines for determining the appropriate treatment pathway. For this project, overweight and obese patients relied on APNs to achieve specific goals and objectives during overweight and obesity management.

The health belief model (HBM), developed by Hochbaum (1952) and expanded by Rosenstock (1974), also supported the development of the intervention procedures of this project. The HBM has several constructs that predict why people will prevent, control, or screen for disease. These constructs include perceived susceptibility, perceived severity, perceived benefits, perceived barriers, cues to action, and self-efficacy. These three constructs: perceived susceptibility, perceived benefits, and perceived barriers, were selected because they were better aligned with the purpose of the project. However, for perceived susceptibility, perceived benefits, and perceived barriers, the literature supports these constructs' validity consistency when translated into practice (Hochbaum, 1952; Rosenstock, 1974). For this project, these constructs were utilized to determine the intent to screen and treat overweight and obese adults using AHA, ACC, and TOS guidelines. This project aims to identify overweight and obese adults' intentions concerning weight loss and obesity risk knowledge after implementing AHA, ACC, and TOS guidelines using HBM constructs.

One of this project's assumptions is that the health belief model is suitable for guiding the APNs in implementing an evidence-based practice guideline. Because many studies have utilized the HBM as a framework, it is assumed that it is supported empirically. Furthermore, the implementation of evidence-based practice guidelines is valid and reliable, as referenced in many studies (Chan et al., 2017; Gomersall, 2017; Slade, 2018). AHA, ACC, and TOS guidelines should be used to ensure the patient understands the seriousness of obesity and its relation to comorbidities.

Significance of the Project

Quality improvement depends on systems and continuous evidence-based interventions that result in measurable improvement in healthcare service and the patient's health status (Melnyk et al., 2017). The PCPs must be prepared to care for two-thirds of the American population suffering from overweight or obesity. According to Simon and Lahiri (2018), evidence-based practice guidelines focus on a five to ten percent weight loss; health benefits for as little as a three percent weight loss. Since primary care setting is often the point of entry for many patients, it should be the primary site to prevent and manage overweight and obesity. The PCPs must take the lead to change the course of the disease. Despite the abundance of high-quality, evidence-based AHA, ACC, and TOS guidelines for treating patients with overweight and obesity, there is a documented gap in practice. According to Jensen et al. (2014), utilization of the AHA, ACC, and TOS guidelines increased weight loss outcomes, CVD, and obesity-risk knowledge. While literature indicated that the AHA, ACC, and TOS guidelines were a choice for managing overweight and obese patients, the project site did not have clinical guidelines or standardized protocols for managing overweight and obesity. There is a lack of information about obesity lifestyle interventions for PCPs in a primary care setting (Jensen et al., 2014). The AHA, ACC, and TOS guidelines recognized that research is needed to understand better and improve the efficiency of overweight and obesity management in a primary care setting (Jensen et al., 2014).

A study by Lopez (2016) used AHA, ACC, and TOS guidelines as a reference to assess the weight and blood pressure changes of adult participants in an outpatient clinic in Texas. The 285 participants that completed the intervention achieved an average weight loss of 1.48% ±3.33. The median weight loss of 1.31±3.3 kg was statistically significant (p=0.001), representing a 0.5±1.29 kg/m2 (*p*=0.001) decrease in overall BMI measurements. The study by Jakicic et al. (2018) showed that Physical activity was inversely associated with weight gain and the incidence of obesity and contributed to additional weight loss when coupled with dietary modification. Relative to the problem identified, It was not known if or to what degree the implementation of AHA, ACC, and TOS guidelines would impact weight, BMI, and obesity risk knowledge compared to current practice among adults with BMI greater than 25 kg/m2. This project sought the best available evidence, personal experience, and patient preference when introducing the evidence-based practice AHA, ACC, and TOS guidelines to APNs. The evidence-based practice AHA, ACC, and TOS guidelines provided the steps to address and treat overweight and obesity at the project site.

The project site was not utilizing any guidelines to assess and treat overweight and obesity until August 2020. The evidence-based guidelines suggest the elements of weight loss lifestyle interventions that have been proven to result in clinically meaningful health benefits for patients. Nevertheless, the guidelines also report the gaps in evidence, such as the need to understand and improve the efficiency of evidence-based weight-loss interventions using the AHA, ACC, and TOS guidelines in a primary care setting. An improvement project was needed to improve lifestyle interventions ' efficiency based on evidence gaps stated in the AHA, ACC, and TOS guidelines. Literature has identified that treating patients using the AHA/ACC/TOS guidelines is a significant factor in weight loss success (Bray et al., 2017). According to Bray et al. (2017), even though there is considerable evidence of effective weight management programs and guidelines for obesity treatment, many PCPs are uncertain of what strategies comprise the most effective weight-loss interventions. This quality improvement project t will consulate the best evidence into a brief intervention to increase APNs' use of AHA, ACC, and TOS guidelines to diagnose and treat obesity and overweight. The first step in treatment is an appropriate screening and diagnosis. Without screening and diagnosis, there will be no plan. Evidence illustrates that despite the recommendation to screen adults for obesity and overweight, the number of individuals diagnosed is low (Hayes et al., 2017).

The project will offer the opportunity to help APNs in the clinic advance the quality of patient care. The completion of this project will provide a step toward closing the gap that currently exists in the literature. It will add quantitatively to practice improvement at the project site with respect to overweight and obesity management, similar to other chronic illnesses in a primary care setting. Moreover, this project's results will offer the stimulus for a further project using the AHA, ACC, and TOS guidelines in the primary care setting to help bridge the current gap. This project will also serve as a baseline for increased interventions provided by APNs and other health care professionals through education and practice. Subsequently, these findings will serve as a reference point for concerned stakeholders concerning health/public policy when considering intervention for overweight and obese adults.

Rationale for Methodology

The methodology selected for the quality improvement project was quantitative. The quantitative method is a strategy that focuses on quantifying the collection and analysis of data. This quantitative method is formed from a deductive approach when the emphasis is placed on the testing of intervention (Porter, 2018). There are two principal aims of quantitative research design, (i) to minimize the effects of other variables (confounders) or the results, which may mask the impact of the intervention or treatment, and (ii) to reduce bias through study design or statistical analysis techniques. This project's quantitative method was used to measure the weight changes, BMI, and obesity risk knowledge after implementing AHA, ACC, and TOS guidelines. After the participants received the intervention, their weight, BMI, and obesity risk knowledge will be compared to baseline weight to determine the effect of the intervention.

The direct practice improvement project's outcome would be identifying how much weight changed and obesity risk knowledge occurred in participants during the project period. The outcome data gathered would present how many changes occurred to support quantitative measures for this direct practice improvement project. The rationale for selecting a quantitative methodology was implementing evidence-based practice AHA, ACC, and TOS guidelines to facilitate overweight and obesity management and analyze the data before and after the intervention using descriptive statistics (Maciejewski, 2020). Therefore, this quantitative methodology was the appropriate methodology for the pre-intervention and post-intervention of the AHA, ACC, and TOS guidelines. A pre and post-intervention chart audit was the appropriate method of collecting data for the project. This quantitative method was significant because it statistically showed the number of participants that improved post-intervention. The project's success will help APNs include AHA, ACC, and TOS guidelines to manage overweight and obese patients at the clinic.

Nature of the Project Design

The selected design for this project was quasi-experimental with pre-intervention and post-intervention data. A quasi-experimental design provides an empirical intervention process to identify an intervention's causal impact on the target population without randomization (Maciejewski, 2020). This quasi-experimental design project used evidence in literature such as overweight and obesity management to assess AHA, ACC, and TOS guidelines' effect to produce positive patient outcomes. Dependent variables are weight, BMI, and obesity risk knowledge. The independent variable is the AHA/ACC/TOS guidelines. This project's quasi-experimental design demonstrated that weight and BMI quantitative measurements were valid predictors of overweight and obesity and subsequent weight loss among participants who received the intervention. The power of quantitative data is its ability to demonstrate changes in obesity and weight management. The data were obtained from direct measurement of BMI, weight, obesity risk knowledge.

Correlation design is a non-experimental research method in which researchers measure two variables and assess the statistical relationship. The variables were not controlled or manipulated; instead, the researcher tried to distinguish the link and degree of association between variables (Regoniel, 2020). A correlational design could also be used for this project to determine if there was an association between the independent and dependent variables. Quasi experimental designs and correlation designs are similar because they are used when manipulating an independent variable is either impossible or unethical (Miller et al., 2020). An important difference between quasi-experimental and correlational research is that quasi-experimental studies involve two or more groups and one independent variable; in contrast, correlational studies involve two or more variables (Miller et al., 2020).

Pre-intervention and post-intervention chart audits were performed to answer part of the clinical question to determine if the independent variables (AHA, ACC, and TOS guidelines) impact the dependent variables (weight, BMI). The ORK tool was also used to determine an increase in obesity risk knowledge after implementing the AHA, ACC, and TOS guidelines by the APNs. The participants were selected via a purposive sampling strategy. This strategy allowed the project manager to select participants by predetermined criteria (Porter, 2018). This project's participants consisted of male and female patients aged 18-64 years who were classified as overweight with a BMI of 25-29.9 kg/m^2 and obese with a BMI of 30 kg/m2 or greater.

The sample size was based on G* power analysis, which indicated that a sample size of 27 patients was appropriate for this project. The G* power analysis allowed for selecting patient-participants purposefully by predetermined criteria (Porter, 2018). The sample size may be too small, and studies may be underpowered to detect effects as small as the desired size (Porter, 2018). The criteria for receiving intervention include Patients receiving care at the project site, patients between age 18 and 64, a patient having BMI greater than 25 kg/m^2, and patients living in central California. Collection of baseline data from the patients' paper chart before the intervention and collecting outcome data from the same patient paper chart after the intervention was completed. Data such as initial weight in pounds and BMI were collected pre-intervention and four weeks post-intervention. The ORK-10 questionnaire was administered to obese patients before the intervention and four weeks after intervention. Quantitative analysis was done using descriptive statistics and Statistical Package for Social Sciences (SPSS) that compared patients' pre-intervention and post-intervention outcomes related to weight, BMI, and obesity risk knowledge. The selected design of quasi-experimental was chosen because the studied variables had a cause and effect association. One variable caused another variable to produce an outcome (Maciejewski, 2020).

Definition of Terms

Some obesity experts are conflicting when defining overweight and obesity to their patients or other healthcare providers. Therefore, terminologies specific to this project were determined. The following terms were defined and operationalized in this project.

AHA/ACC/TOS Guidelines

The AHA, ACC, and TOS guidelines refer to step-by-step educational instructions considered the standard of care for managing overweight and obesity in the primary care setting (Bays et al., 2019).

Advanced Practice Nurses (APNs)

APNs are registered nurses with additional training and education such as a master's degree, post-master's certificate, or practice-focused doctor of nursing practice degree that allows them to function independently in a healthcare organization (Leary & MacLaine, 2019).

Body Mass Index

BMI refers to a person's classification by dividing weight in kilograms by the square of their height in meters (kg/m^2; Bays et al., 2019).

Class I Obesity

Class I obesity refers to a BMI of 30 kg/m^2 to 34.9 kg/m^2 (Jensen et al., 2014).

Class II obesity.

Class II obesity is when an individual's BMI is 35 kg/m^2 to 39.9 kg/m^2 (Bays et al., 2019).

Class III Obesity

Class III obesity is when an individual's BMI is equal to or greater than 40 kg/m^2 (Bays et al., 2019).

Obesity

Obesity is an abnormal or excessive fat accumulation that may impair health (Shahadan et al., 2019). An individual with a BMI greater than or equal to 30 kg/m^2 is considered obese (Jensen et al., 2014).

Overweight

Overweight refers to a BMI of 25 kg/m^2 - 29.9 kg/m^2 Bays et al., 2019).

Weight-Loss Outcome

A weight-loss outcome refers to a weight loss of 2%-5% of the initial weight (Bays et al., 2019).

Assumptions, Limitations, and Delimitations

Assumptions were made in the development of this project:

1. It was assumed that participants responded to the survey truthfully. It was believed that all respondents would answer ORK-10 surveys honestly because anonymity and confidentiality were established.
2. It was assumed that the sample was representative of the project site patient population necessary to make inferences. Therefore, according to the power analysis calculation, this project will need a minimum of 27 participants to provide enough data to support the project's validity.
3. It was assumed that overweight and obese patients would abide by the recommended interventions. Obese patients who were consistent with treatment lost weight if they had more structured diets and committed to their exercise routines and follow-up (Bray et al., 2017).

4. It was assumed that APNs screened all participating patients for inclusion in the project based on the BMI. The charts for those patients who met the inclusion criteria were reviewed. The primary investigator has presented that participants for the practice improvement project would be included in the project if their starting BMI is >25 kg/m^2.
5. It was assumed that patients' charts were reviewed retrospectively, represented overweight and obese patients enrolled for the project, and requested weight loss intervention.
6. It was assumed that patients enrolled in the project provided valid information concerning obesity risk knowledge. The participants should be an understanding of the role obesity plays in many diseases. The participants who do not perceive themselves as overweight or obese may be less likely to try to lose weight, putting themselves at risk for developing obesity-related chronic disease (Bray et al., 2017).

Limitations are the characteristics of design or methodology that impacted or influenced the interpretations of the finding from the project. The limitations for the project include:

1. The APNs were instructed to exclude patients presented as a walk-in for urgent care for needs, those younger than 17 and older than 64, and individuals who were not patients set at the project site. Age was a limiting factor as many overweight and obese patients are over 18 years. This age group was chosen to get an adequate sample size.
2. Participants were volunteering to participate in the project with minimal intention

to change starting weight; participation may be based on the intention to support or not support the primary investigator to complete the practice improvement project.

3. The patients' attitude toward obesity management may affect the outcome. There are limited opportunities for success if the patient believes that nothing can permanently manage their weight. Additionally, some obese patients have no desire to make changes or lose weight.
4. Time to complete the project is a limiting factor and may not represent the effect of a weight management program in the primary care practice setting. A more extended period for weight management may provide different results due to personal factors affecting participation.

Delimitations are things that the investigator controls, such as the project's location, population and sample, and data collection tools. The following delimitations were accepted for the project:

1. Four-week duration of the project's treatment, which led to minimal data on health outcomes. The pre and post-intervention data collected was subjected to bias related to the small sample size. The project occurred during periods when several providers worked fewer hours due to pandemics, resulting in shorter office hours and fewer patient visits.
2. The project was implemented in one primary care setting, which limited the result's generalizability. The participants for the project were selected from the primary care setting in central California; therefore, they did not represent the entirety of California.

3. Participants who answered the ORK-10 questionnaire were recruited from a single site and were selected with inclusion and exclusion criteria to complete the survey, limiting the results' generalizability.
4. The project manager anticipated that the direct practice improvement project might not provide immediate outcomes or changes in patient weight if the same intervention was implemented on larger samples for a more extended period.
5. The APNs provided intervention to all patients during their routine visits. APNs informed the patients with BMI less than 25 kg/m^2 to maintain their weight and have a yearly weight check, and those with BMI greater than 25 kg/m^2 were treated based on the evidence-based AHA/ACC/TOS guidelines (Bays et al., 2019; Jensen et al., 2014).
6. When APNs provided intervention to patients with normal weight, the patients received equal treatment. The APNs implemented the evidence-based AHA/ACC/TOS guidelines on the patients who had appointments but not as a walk-in for urgent care.

Summary and Organization of the Remainder of the Project

Overweight and obesity are among the most significant healthcare issues in the United States (CDC, 2018). The overweight and obesity management guidelines for adults in primary care settings were published by Jensen et al. (2014). Obesity has become a chronic condition that requires intervention by APNs using AHA/ACC/TOS guidelines to decrease mortality. The quantitative quasi-experimental project sought to determine if there was a reduction in weight, BMI, and increase in obesity risk knowledge among adults with BMI greater than 25 kg/m^2 after intervention utilizing evidence-based practice AHA/ACC/TOS guidelines by APNs. The patient needs to develop self-management behaviors to sustain the change over a lifetime as recommended by the AHA/ACC/TOS guidelines. The application TGA and HBM guided this project.

Due to the growing prevalence of obesity and the associated comorbidities, treating overweight and obesity has become a priority concern in primary care settings (Jensen. et al., 2014). Overweight and obesity management guidelines published by AHA/ACC/TOS guide PCPs in identifying those at risk for obesity and providing treatment outlined in the guidelines (Jensen et al., 2014). The following chapters will continue the project aimed at introducing the AHA/ACC/TOS guidelines at the project site and how they performed in reducing weight, BMI, and increase obesity risk knowledge.

Chapter 1 discussed the introduction and background for the general purpose of the project. It included the project's background of the prevalence of overweight and obesity in adults. The problem statement was presented along with the specific clinical question and how it advances scientific knowledge. The project's significance, the rationale for the methodology, and the nature of the research design were also discussed. The key terms discussed in this study were defined both theoretically and operationally. Assumptions of the project were explored, including the limitations and delimitations. Chapter 1 concluded with the project's summary and organization.

Chapter 2 presents a literature review that evaluates whether the implementation of the AHA, ACC, and TOS guidelines would impact patient outcomes of weight, BMI, and obesity risk knowledge. The literature review outlines the themes relating to managing overweight and obese adults in a primary care setting. Theories applicable to the project are discussed. Chapter 3 presents the methodology, design, population and sample selection, and instrumentation of the direct practice improvement project. The validity and reliability of the instrument and how data were collected and analyzed are discussed. The ethical considerations and limitations of the project conclude the discussion in Chapter 3. The statistical analysis of the findings using tables and figures is presented in Chapter 4. Finally, Chapter 5 presents a summary of the project, its findings, and conclusions. Theoretical, practical, and future implications conclude Chapter 5.

Chapter 2: Literature Review

Obesity and overweight are linked to an increased risk for many diseases. Epidemiologists recognized the link between obesity and adverse health effects, identifying obesity as a risk factor or exposure to many illnesses. Overweight and obesity are preventable health problems (Bays et al., 2019). Obesity persists for multiple reasons; it is not merely an issue of low self-control concerning foods or a lack of motivation to move. There are specific biochemical adaptations that characterize obesity as a chronic disease (Nourian et al., 2020). Only 26% of primary care providers provide counseling or treatment routinely (Hayes, 2019). One contributing factor stands out: during annual well-visits, less than 50% of obese adults reported that their primary care physician addressed weight management (Hayes, 2019). Primary care providers are positioned to treat patients with overweight and obesity, influencing and impacting the course of the disease. Despite the numerous clinical practice guidelines, patients are not receiving the care they require until late in the disease process (Granara & Laurent, 2017). According to Hayes (2019), even though clinical practice guidelines are available, the under-treatment of overweight and obesity in primary care persists. This direct practice improvement project introduced AHA, ACC, and TOS guidelines to APNs to reference overweight and obesity management in primary care settings to improve patient outcomes. AHA, ACC and TOS guidelines are evidence-based developed by expert panels for PCPs to manage overweight and obesity and reduce cardiovascular risk (Jensen et al., 2014). The evidence-based guidelines suggested the elements of weight-loss interventions that have been proven to result in clinically meaningful health benefits for patients. Nevertheless, the guidelines also report the gaps in evidence, such as understanding and improving overweight and obesity management in adults.

The literature review was divided into three themes: obesity-related risk and knowledge with the following subthemes (cancer, T2DM, and CVD), the second theme was the treatment of overweight and obesity, the subthemes (diet and physical activity), the final theme was a clinical guideline for treating overweight and obesity; the subthemes (AHA, ACC, and TOS guidelines, American Association of Clinical Endocrinologists and the American College of Endocrinology (AACE-ACE), and OMA). A comprehensive literature review was performed utilizing the following databases: Google Scholar, Cumulative Index to Nursing and Allied Health Literature (CINAHL), and PubMed. Search terms were used independently and in various combinations with the operators OR and. The review was limited to the most recent five years of peer-reviewed or scholarly journals. The search keywords included: *AHA, ACC, and TOS, Agency for Healthcare Research and Quality (AHRQ) Tool 2 Audit Form AHRQ Tool 2 Audit Form, Obesity risk knowledge (ORK-10), overweight, obesity, primary care, King's theory of goal attainment, health belief model.*

Adult overweight and obesity continue to rise despite the availability of evidence-based clinical guidelines. According to the Clinical Guidelines on the Identification, Evaluation, and Treatment of Overweight and Obesity in Adults, overweight is defined as a condition when people have a BMI of 25 kg/m^2 – 29.99 kg/m^{2,} and obesity is consistent with a BMI equal or greater than 30 kg/m^2. The APNs at the project site did not have clinical guidelines for managing overweight or obesity, putting patients at risk for obesity-related diseases. APNs and other PCPs could address overweight and obesity, just like other health conditions. Evidence had shown that PCPs did not consistently discuss overweight and obesity during their regular office visits (Kahan, 2018). According to Hayes et al. (2017), patients were most likely to make an effort towards weight loss when receiving counseling from their PCPs. The project goal is to introduce evidence-based practice AHA, ACC, and TOS guidelines to reduce weight and BMI and increase obesity risk knowledge among overweight and obese patients at the primary project site. The following chapters continue the project to introduce the AHA, ACC, and TOS guidelines to APNs at the project site.

Theoretical Foundations

Two theories were integrated into this project to impact overweight and obesity in a primary care clinic. The theories included Imogene King's theory of goal attainment (TGA) and the health belief model (HBM). The TGA was chosen for this project based on the affiliation formed between a nurse and a patient. The TGA applied the nursing process with interacting systems focusing on assessment, diagnosis, planning, and evaluation to identify and treat overweight and obese adults. The HBM was selected because the framework aligned with the project's purpose and can support the search for obesity-related risk and knowledge.

Imogene King's Theory of Goal Attainment

The TGA was developed by Imogene King in the early 1960s to describe an interpersonal relationship between a nurse and a patient to help the patient learns to develop and attain specific goals. The several assumptions of TGA are rooted in individuals, communication, and nursing (King, 1992). Individuals are seen as social beings that can reason, manipulate situations, and act in purposeful manners (King,

1992). The assumption on communication is that nurse-client interactions are affected by nurse and client involvement (King, 1992). According to TGA, the client has the right to knowledge, participates in care decisions, and denies or accepts treatment, and that the client and nurse may not gear toward the same goal (King, 1997). King defined nursing as human care through perception, judgment, thoughts, and relationships with clients (King, 1997). The TGA also described nursing as the setting of care where the nurse-client interaction is established to help the client or groups attain, maintain, or die respectfully (King, 2007).

This project involved the nurse and patient working together, communicating information, and setting desired mutually accepted and congruent goals. A patient developed goals to manage obesity. The APN s complete assessment, diagnosis, planning, and evaluation based on patient goals. The APNs communicate the treatment plan to attain a state of well-being for the patient. The TGA has four meta-paradigm levels within her theory: health, person, environment, and nursing (King, 2007). Human beings are unique and can make decisions, think, feel, and perceive. According to King (2007), each human being has three central needs: health information, preventative measures, and assistance with self-care deficits. Health is life experiences that are a continuous alteration and adaptation to the environment's stressors (King, 2007). The setting is the realm of human interactions that allow nurses to perceive the clients and adapt to the environment's stressors (King, 2007). Stressors can either be internal or external, and humans can adjust to stressors and the continuous changes (King, 2007).

The TGA theory implies that assessment, diagnosis, planning, and implementation correlate to perception, judgment, and action (King, 2007). Interaction and transaction relate to evaluation as feedback described the exchange of information throughout the relationship between the APNs and the overweight and obese patients. The nurse's function for this project was to use the nursing process to plan, implement, and evaluate the outcome. The TGA applied the nursing process with interacting systems, addressing the interaction and feedback between nurses and patients (King, 1997).

The scholarly project examined specific aspects of the interaction between APNs and patients, independent of AHA, ACC, and TOS guidelines for determining the appropriate treatment pathway. King's transaction process model demonstrated the interaction between the APN and the patient in overweight and obesity. This model reflected the nursing process from both the APN and the client standpoint. The TGA reflected the nursing process from the APNs and the patients working together to communicate information, set goals together, and take actions to achieve weight loss outcomes

The effectiveness of interventions based on the TGA was demonstrated in a quasi-experimental, longitudinal, randomized study to examine how people with T2DM can improve care and adherence to treatment in a primary care setting (Araujo et al., 2018). Their participant sample consisted of 60 participants with diabetes, divided into intervention and control groups. The intervention group received the nursing consultation based on the TGA, while the control group received standard of care. The intervention group had a significant adherence of the patients to the study's goals, and the control group improved some aspects of the treatment. The project manager concludes that using the TGA for this project improved positive aspects of adherence to weight loss intervention and improved quality of life.

Health Belief Model

The HBM is a psychological model that attempts to explain and predict health behaviors (Rosenstock, 1974). The primary focus is on the attitudes and beliefs of individuals. The HBM has several constructs that explain or predict why people will prevent, control, or screen for disease (Rosenstock, 1974). The assumptions of this project are parallel to the ones of the HBM. According to Rosenstock (1974), the HBM is based on the assumptions that a person will take a health-related action (i.e., participate in a weight management program) if that person: (a) feels that a negative health condition (i.e., obesity-related risk such as T2DM, CVD or cancer) can be avoided; (b) has a positive expectation that by taking a recommended action (i.e., eating a low-calorie diet, and increase physical activity will be effective at preventing obesity-related risk.); and (c) believes that recommended health action can be achieved successfully (i.e., able to schedule for assessment and screening for obesity-related risk).

The HBM addressed the effects of beliefs on health and the decision process in making behavioral changes. The theory asserts that health enhancement behavior was influenced by a person's perception of threat caused by health conditions (Rosenstock, 1974). The model has several constructs that explain or predict why people will prevent, control, or screen for disease (Rosenstock, 1974). The six concepts of HBM were defined as follows:

Perceived Susceptibility. Perceived susceptibility refers to the likelihood of getting a disease or condition. Thus, the HBM predicts that individuals who perceive that they are susceptible to disease will engage in behaviors that would help reduce the risk of developing the disease (Rosenstock, 1974). The concept of perceived susceptibility implied that if overweight or obese patients perceived a threat to developing obesity-related risk for T2DM, they were more likely to be involved in behavior modification.

Perceived Severity. Perceived severity refers to the feeling of the seriousness of contracting the disease or leaving it untreated. The HBM suggests that the more serious individuals perceive a health problem, the more likely they will engage in behaviors to prevent it from occurring or reduce its severity (Rosenstock, 1974). An individual believed that the adverse effects of becoming overweight or obese could cause serious health consequences; the person would be more likely to engage in an intervention to reduce obesity-related risk.

Perceived Benefit. Perceived benefits refer to an individual's assessment of the value or efficacy of engaging in a health-promoting behavior to decrease a disease's risk. The HBM proposed that the more benefits individuals perceived that a particular action would have regarding a perceived threat, the more likely they would engage in that behavior regardless of the effectiveness of the action (Rosenstock, 1974). Overweight and obese patients who did not believe that a sedentary lifestyle increased overweight would not be involved in any interventions to prevent obesity-related risks. An individual who believed that there was no association between unhealthy eating and weight gain was unlikely to assume healthier eating patterns to prevent obesity-related risk.

Perceived Barrier. Perceived barriers refer to potential complications involved with a particular health action. These factors act as impediments to undertaking recommended behaviors. The HBM suggests that the perceived benefits must outweigh the perceived barriers for behavior change to occur (Rosenstock, 1974). For example, obese patients could present several barriers to participating in a weight management program, resulting in weight gain and chronic diseases.

Cues to Action. Cues to action refer to the internal or external cues that prompt the action. The HBM theorizes that a cue, or trigger, is necessary for promoting engagement in health-promoting behaviors. Internal cues can be physiological such as pain, whereas external cues can be an event or a billboard sign (Rosenstock, 1974). For example, suppose a family member was recently diagnosed with T2DM due to severe obesity. In that case, the other family members are more likely to have the intent to start exercising and eat healthy to prevent obesity.

Self-Efficacy. Self-efficacy refers to an individual's perception of their competence to perform a behavior successfully. The HBM recognizes that confidence in the individual's ability to effect change in outcomes is crucial to health behavior change (Rosenstock, 1974). Overweight and obese patients might not want to adapt to new behavior due to culture, illness, or economic status; however, there were chances for the intervention to be achieved.

The three constructs, perceived susceptibility, perceived benefits, and perceived barriers for this project, were aligned with the purpose of the project. They correlated well with the model's assumptions. However, for perceived susceptibility, perceived benefits, and perceived barriers, the literature supports the consistency in construct validity when translated into practice Rosenstock 1974. (Rosenstock, 1974). For this project, perceived susceptibility, perceived benefits, and perceived barriers were utilized to determine the intent of obese adults regarding obesity risk knowledge. An individual identifies whether obesity is at risk for developing T2DM, CVD, or cancer. Nevertheless, all of these three select constructs have a direct impact on the likelihood of a behavior.

Soliman et al. (2018) used a quasi-experimental design to evaluate the effect of the application of HBM among 117 youth who were at high risk for obesity in the West Bank. A self-administered questionnaire was used for anthropometric measurements and levels of risk for obesity. Soliman et al. (2018) found a significant difference between students' knowledge and their practices regarding obesity, healthy food, and exercises pre-application & post-application of HBM. The recommendation was to incorporate HBM in routine practice, especially with those at risk for obesity and other related illnesses (Soliman et al., 2018).

The TGA and HBM were used as models to implement this direct practice improvement project. Behavior change could affect overweight and obese patients who could have better health outcomes by engaging in health promotion practices such as healthy eating and physical activity. These frameworks provided a foundation for understanding weight loss and obesity risk knowledge and developing an effective intervention to improve clinical outcomes at the project site.

The AHA, ACC, and TOS guidelines developed to manage overweight and obesity in adults are supported for these frameworks to assess the patient's behavior to make lifestyle changes to achieve weight loss outcomes (Jensen et al., 2014). Regardless of the participant's weight, either prevention or weight-loss counseling should occur among all patients. According to (Bays et al., 2019), the health risk awareness due to overweight and obesity should be advice by PCPs to patients and provide counseling about weight loss and lifestyle changes. The expected outcomes were increased in intent to treat, leading to APNs utilizing the evidence-based ACA, ACC, and TOS guidelines to manage overweight and obesity. Ultimately, the goal was to reach permanent practice change with ongoing intention to treat and successfully sustained weight reduction in a primary care setting at the project site.

Review of the Literature

Chan et al. (2017) reported that obesity prevention and management using the AHA, ACC, and TOS guidelines to be the most recent and comprehensive clinical guideline for treating overweight and obese adults in primary care settings. A literature review revealed no studies addressing adult overweight or obesity by APNs in the primary care setting. According to Noble and Smith (2018), the purpose of the literature review is to summarize the knowledge around a specific question and provide recommendations that can support health professionals and organizations make decisions about a particular intervention. This project is unique because it examined the effect of using the AHA, ACC, and TOS guidelines to recognize and treat adult overweight and obesity in a primary care setting. In the United States, data reporting the management of overweight and obese patients in primary care settings showed that adherence to evidence-based landmark clinical guidelines was not consistently practiced. The reason for not adhering to clinical guidelines was a lack of awareness (Fruh et al., 2019; Turner et al., 2018). The importance of using evidence-based guidelines is critical for APNs to assess and treat overweight and obesity to prevent developing obesity-related risks such as T2DM, CVD, and cancers (Hayes, 2019).

This chapter includes three major themes and their subthemes related to the management of overweight and obesity using clinical guidelines. The first theme was obesity-related risk and complication with the following subthemes: cancer, T2DM, and CVD. The second theme was the overweight and obesity intervention. The subthemes were AHA, ACC, and TOS guidelines, the American Association of Clinical Endocrinologists, and the American College of Endocrinology (AACE-ACE), OMA, diet, and physical activity.

Obesity-Related Risks and Complications

There should be an understanding of the role obesity plays in many diseases. Some individuals often did not perceive themselves as overweight or obese and may be less likely to try to lose weight, putting themselves at risk for developing obesity-related chronic disease (Bray et al., 2017). Poor dietary habits and physical inactivity were obesity risk factors (Bray et al., 2017).

Cancer. Overweight and obesity were established risk factors for cancer and other chronic diseases (Arnold et al., 2017). Excess weight has become the leading risk factor for disease burden in high-income countries and has been offsetting or surpassing the decreasing disease burden attributable to tobacco smoking (Arnold et al., 2017).

Baumeister et al. (2021) used a prospective cohort to examine the association of indicators of obesity and body fat distribution with ovarian cancer risk. The 566,398 postmenopausal women completed questionnaires. Six months after completing the baseline questionnaire, a second questionnaire was mailed to participants who did not have a self-reported height, weight, waist circumference, and colon cancer diagnosis. Cox proportional hazards regression was used for estimating adjusted hazard ratios (HRs) and 95% confidence intervals (CIs) for overall ovarian cancer and ovarian cancer subtypes. The mean (SD) age at baseline was 61.8 years. During a follow-up of 12 years, participants reported 683 ovarian cancers (Baumeister et al., 2021). The finding showed the HRs for overall ovarian cancer per SD increment in BMI, waist circumference, hip circumference, waist-hip ratio, and waist-height ratio were: 0.98 (95% CI 0.88–1.10), 1.08 (95% CI 0.91–1.27), 1.06 (95% CI 0.90–1.25), 1.03 (95% CI 0.89–1.21), and 1.08 (95% CI 0.92–1.27) respectively (Baumeister et al., 2021). Neither body mass index nor other anthropometric measurements were associated with ovarian cancer risk (Baumeister et al., 2021). The results supported the hypothesis that there were no associations between obesity and body fat distribution and the risk of ovarian cancer. This study's strength was the large sample size and long-term follow-up. The weakness was self-administered questionnaires which could h have posed the potential measurement error. Future studies on body weight and body fatness changes over the life course were recommended.

Wilkinson et al. (2020) used a nonexperimental exploratory study to examine 50 adult obese patients' attitudes regarding their risk for developing endometrial cancer. The investigators used a 5-point Likert scale for data collection. The first three questions were designed to ascertain whether that patient understood obesity as a disease and determined whether patients felt obesity was a risk factor for endometrial cancer. The participants were assessed for their understanding of the benefits of weight-loss interventions. Participants were la evaluated for their willingness to consider diet, medication, and metabolic surgery as an alternative to surgery in treating endometrial cancer. Wilkinson et al. (2020) found that weight loss treatments were considered an acceptable option for obese patients instead of surgery; 53% of participants believed that obesity could cause cancer. Perhaps the most important finding from this questionnaire was that 84.5% (38/45) of patients would prefer a combined weight loss approach over conventional hysterectomy if weight loss were proven to be equally efficacious in treating endometrial cancer. The strength of this survey was the response rate (45/50). The limitation was the sample size; the study examined women in a primary care setting; therefore, it could not generalize to all people and other locations. Further research was needed to evaluate the difference in perception between younger patients with obesity and endometrial cancer.

Hall et al. (2019) used cross-sectional to explore the relationship between weight status and perceived risk of colorectal (CRC) and breast cancers by race and ethnicity. The National Health Interview Survey (NHIS) was the principal source of information representative sample of the civilian noninstitutionalized US population of females 18 years and over without any reported history of a cancer diagnosis. A questionnaire was administered to each family within the sampled household in 2005, 2010, and 2015. All analyses were conducted using SAS version 9.3 and SAS-callable SUDAAN version 11.0. A test of the trend was performed using logistic regression to detect CRC and breast cancer risk perception changes. Risk perception for both cancers did not change significantly between 2005 and 2010; however, breast and CRC risk perception declined slightly in 2015 compared to 2005, and this difference was statistically significant ($p < 0.05$). Non-Hispanic White women with obesity were more likely to perceive themselves at risk for CRC than their normal and overweight counterparts. Neither non-Hispanic Black nor Hispanic women with obesity perceived themselves at risk for CRC. In comparison, non-Hispanic white women and Hispanic women with obesity and those overweight were more likely to perceive the risk of breast cancer than their normal-weight counterparts. In contrast, non-Hispanic black women did not perceive a higher risk of breast cancer at any weight (Hall et al., 2019). The strengths of this study were the diversity of the sample and the duration of the study. The limitation of the study was the use of self-reported data that might lead to misclassification of BMI. The authors recommended educating women about the risk posed by excess weight for some cancers and their actions to reduce their risk.

An observational study by Welti et al. (2017) investigated if weight fluctuation had a risk factor for postmenopausal breast cancer (PBC) among 80943 women between ages 50 and 79. Welti et al. (2017) hypothesized that weight fluctuation increased the risk of developing PBC. The data collection was based on interviews and self-administered questionnaires. Descriptive statistics and ANOVA were used for baseline data analysis. Hazard ratio (HR) and 95% confidence intervals were used to determine the association between weight fluctuation and breast, endometrial and colorectal cancer incidence. The weight fluctuation was measured using a linear regression model for the participant's BMI recorded. Women with a positive slope from this regression were defined as weight gainers. Welti et al. (2017) noted that a total of 7,464 women were diagnosed with cancers (5,564 breast cancers, 788 endometrial cancers, and 1,290 colorectal cancers). When compared with women with stable weight, Welti et al. (2017) found that weight gain was significantly associated with the risk of breast cancer (HR 1.11, 1.03-120) and endometrial cancer (HR 1.23, 1.01-1.49). The results of this study stressed the importance of maintaining weight loss and avoiding weight fluctuation to prevent the risk of postmenopausal cancers. The strength of the study was the use of a national database and the large sample size. The limitation was the self-reported weight, which could have introduced recall bias.

Steele et al. (2017) used a correlational, cross-sectional study with a convenience sample of 143 obese adults to assess their perception of developing cancer. The researchers used bivariate correlational analysis for the study. Regression analysis was carried out to identify any predictive relationship between the variables. The findings partially were highly correlated ($p < 0.05$) to fear and developing cancer. Perception of risk was much lower than actual risk. Fear was not predictive of weight reduction ($p = 0.81$). The study results indicated that obese adults do not recognize their increased risk for cancer, so they are less likely to be involved in weight loss programs. The study's recommendations for obese adults must be educated on their risk to be adequately equipped to make an informed decision regarding weight loss.

Luo et al. (2017) evaluated associations between weight changes among 161,808 women ages 50 to 79 years with endometrial cancer in the Women's Health Initiative (WHI) observational study. The participants were recruited at 40 clinical centers throughout the United States. Weight change between baseline and three-year follow-up was calculated from the measured weights grouped into stable weight, weight loss, or weight gain. The women were asked to complete a questionnaire regarding weight gain or weight loss during a three-year follow–up. Endometrial cancer occurrences were initially identified by self-report from questionnaires administered annually. Cox proportional hazards regression models were used to evaluate the relationship between weight change and the incidence of endometrial cancer. The women with weight loss significantly lower endometrial cancer risk (HR, 0.71; 95% CI, 0.54 to 0.95). The association was strongest among obese women with intentional weight loss (HR, 0.44; 95% CI, 0.25 to 0.78). Weight gain of more than 10 pounds was associated with higher endometrial cancer risk than women with stable weight. The Strengths of the study was the large prospective design with long-term follow-up (Luo et al., 2017). The limitation of the study was the inclusion of only postmenopausal women; therefore, it could not be generalized to the entire population of women.

In summary, cancers were linked in the literature as risk factors to obesity. The review's findings indicated that as individual weight increases, the risk of developing some cancers increases (Luo et al., 2017; Steele et al., 2017; Welti et al., 2017; Wilkinson et al., 2020). One study found that obesity or high BMI was not associated with ovarian cancer risk (Baumeister et al., 2021). Hall et al. (2019) found that some obese women did not perceive a higher risk of breast cancer at any weight. The results of this study stressed the importance of education on awareness of obesity-related cancers and the risk associated with higher BMI.

Type 2 Diabetes Mellitus. Overweight and obesity are costly on multiple levels. At the individual level, it leads to a multitude of metabolic changes, which increase the risk of developing chronic diseases. A chronic condition associated with overweight and obese adults was T2DM (Kinlen et al., 2018). People with a BMI greater than 30 kg/m2 were 80 times more likely to develop T2DM than people with lower BMI (Kinlen et al., 2018).

Schnurr et al. (2020) used a case-cohort study to examine the association of obesity, genetic predisposition, and unfavorable lifestyle with T2DM, which involved a sample of 4,729 adult men and women. The mean age of the participants was 56.1 years. Approximately 21.8% of the participants were obese, while 43.0% were overweight. Lifestyle was assessed by a lifestyle score composed of smoking, alcohol consumption, physical activity, and diet. Schnurr et al. (2020) used Prentice-weighted Cox proportional-hazards models to test the genetic, obesity, and lifestyle score associations with incident T2DM. Obesity and unfavorable lifestyle were associated with a higher risk for T2DM regardless of genetic predisposition ($p > 0.05$ for obesity and lifestyle interaction). The effect of obesity on T2DM risk (HR 5.81 [95% CI 5.16, 6.55]) was high, whereas the impact of genetic risk (HR 2.00 [95% CI 1.76, 2.27]) and unfavorable lifestyle (HR 1.18 [95% CI 1.06, 1.30]) was relatively low. Individuals with obesity and an unfavorable lifestyle are at greater risk of T2DM regardless of their genetic risk. Average body weight is crucial in the prevention of T2DM regardless of genetic. The results suggest that T2DM prevention by weight management and healthy lifestyle prevention are critical across all genetic risk groups. The strength of the study was the long follow-up period. Information on lifestyle was collected before type 2 diabetes diagnosis, ensuring that recall bias did not influence the results. As a limitation, the analysis was performed in a European genetic ancestry population and cannot be generalized to other ancestry groups.

Ko et al. (2020) used a retrospective cohort study to examine the health screening using data from 5,590,120 men and 4,102 523 women between the age of 20 and 79 who were followed up for two years for 10 years to identify adults who did not have a diagnosis of T2DM. Physical activity questionnaires about weekly exercise frequency were used to define low physical activity (LPA), moderate physical activity (MPA), and high physical activity (HPA). Relative risk (RR) was calculated using Cox analysis. The statistical analysis system (SAS) version 9.4 and one-way ANOVA were used for data analysis. Among men, 82.1% had LPA, 10.7% had MPA, and 7.2% had HPA, whereas

84.9%, 8.1%, and 7.0% of women had LPA, MPA, and HPA, respectively. The BMI was the lowest in the HPA group for both men and women, and in the HPA groups, the proportions of men and women with normal BMIs were 82.1% and 74.3%, respectively (*p*<0.001). Diabetes incidence rates were 14.8% in overweight men, 20.0% in men with obesity, 17.9% in overweight women, and 22.7% in women with obesity (Ko et al., 2020). The strength of the study was the large sample with long-term follow-up. Limitation includes lack of family history, nutrition status, or lifestyle surveys. Ko et al. (2020) recommended further study on the prevention of obesity and complications of T2DM through post-diabetes tracking and physical activity, which will lead to better management of obesity and T2DM.

Maskarinec et al. (2019) used a retrospective design to evaluate obesity and T2DM, and breast cancer risk. Maskarinec et al. (2019) analyzed 29,818 Japanese women using cancer registries and vital records for assessing BMI and diabetes status in association with breast cancer. The researchers used Cox regression to estimate hazard ratios (HR) and 95% confidence intervals (CI) for BMI and diabetes status. According to Maskarinec et al., 2019, diabetes prevalence increased from 2.6% to 5.3% and 7.5% from the first to the second and third data collection. During 27 years of follow-up, 703 women had developed breast cancer, and 31 had been diagnosed with diabetes. Diabetes diagnosis was not significantly associated with breast cancer incidence; the respective HRs for overweight and obesity were 1.61 (95% CI 1.34–1.93) and 2.04 (95% CI 1.40–2.97). The result indicated that increased BMI was significantly associated with breast cancer risk but not T2DM among Japanese women (Maskarinec et al., 2019). This study's strength was the large sample size and long-term follow-up; the weakness was self-administered questionnaires.

A cross-sectional study and retrospective cohort design involved 1263 women with gestational diabetes (GDM) and 705 with non-GDM were examined to determine the effects of GDM, pre-pregnancy, and postpartum BMI (Fan et al., 2019). The researchers assessed a history of GDM, pre-pregnancy overweight, early postpartum overweight, high body fat, and abdominal obesity using questionnaires (Fan et al., 2019). The analyses were performed using a *t*-test, chi-square, and SPSS version 25.0. Cox hazards regression was used to estimate independent and combined effects of a history of GDM and pre-pregnancy BMI on the risks of diabetes and hyperglycemia. The researchers reported odds ratios at different postpartum BMI levels (<24, 24–27.9, and ≥ 28 kg/m^2) were 1.00, 2.80, and 8.08 for diabetes ($P < 0.001$), and 1.00, 2.10, and 4.42 for hyperglycemia ($P < 0.001$), respectively (Fan et al., 2019). Women with high body fat (≥31.9%) had a 2.7–6.9-fold higher odds ratio for diabetes or hyperglycemia (Fan et al., 2019). The researchers concluded that women with pre-pregnancy overweight and postpartum overweight had an increased risk of postpartum diabetes and hyperglycemia. The strength of the study was the large sample size. Several limitations were using two different studies (cross-sectional study and a retrospective cohort study design); some women were not screened until three months postpartum, resulting in recall bias.

Fitzpatrick and Steven (2017) used a retrospective study to examine the rates of (BMI) screening, T2DM diagnosis, and weight management counseling in the U.S. from 2008 to 2013 with 14,143 overweight, and sample from a total of 55,608 primary care visits. The National Ambulatory Medical Care Survey visit-level data for adults 18 and over with a primary care visit during survey years 2008–2009, 2010–2011, and 2012–2013 were included in the analyses using Statistical analysis System (SAS) version 9.3. Study outcomes included percent of visits with BMI screening, obesity diagnosis, and weight counseling. Fitzpatrick and Steven (2017) compared survey years on these outcomes using 2008–2009 as the reference and examined patient and practice-level predictors. Analyses were conducted from 2015 to early 2017. BMI screening significantly increased between 2008–2009 and 2012–2013 from 54% to 73% (OR = 1.75, 95% CI 1.28–2.41); however, percent of visits with T2DM diagnosis remained low at < 30%. Weight management counseling during visits significantly declined from 33% to 21% between 2008 2009 and 2012 2013 (OR = 0.62, 95% CI 0.41–0.92). Despite emerging recommendations and policies, from 2008 to 2013, obesity management in primary care remained low. Fitzpatrick and Steven (2017) recommended that identifying practical strategies to manage overweight and obesity and implement evidence-based treatment in primary care should be a high priority for healthcare providers to prevent T2DM.

Hite et al. (2018) used a quantitative method with a survey design to examine the screening for T2DM and identifying BMI as obesity among 206 primary care providers. Hite et al. (2018) hypothesized that the participants would have difficulty diagnosing and managing overweight and obesity and diagnosing T2DM. Another hypothesis was that providers' system-related barriers might interfere with helping patients manage their weight. Hite et al. (2018) found that comfort was the most barrier identified ($p<0.001$). About 6.4% of participants felt uncomfortable discussing the patient's weight, and 4.2%

believed that the patient would feel stigmatized by discussing the topic (Hite et al., 2018). The strength of this study is the significant response rate. One of the limitations is that only 5% of participants were African American, limiting the generalization. The study did include other options for obesity management, such as referral to a dietitian, physiotherapy, or support group (Hite et al., 2018).

In summary, all studies reported similar findings that individuals with obesity are at risk for developing T2DM (Fan et al., 2019; Hite et al., 2018; Ko et al., 2020; Schnurr et al., 2020). The women were three times more likely than men to develop T2DM (Ko et al., 2020). Obesity was considered the most modifiable risk factor for T2DM; therefore, increased physical activity level would slow the disease's development. One study did not find an association between obesity and T2DM (Maskarinec et al., 2019). The result indicated that increased BMI was significantly associated with breast cancer risk but not T2DM among Japanese women (Maskarinec et al., 2019). The finding from four studies suggests that identifying practical strategies to manage overweight and obesity and implementing evidence-based treatment in primary care should be a high priority for healthcare providers to prevent T2DM (Fan et al., 2019; Hite et al., 2018; Ko et al., 2020; Schnurr et al., 2020).

Cardiovascular Disease. The adverse effects of obesity on CVD health manifest as the accelerated progression of atherosclerosis, higher rates of ventricular remodeling, and a higher risk of associated diseases, including stroke, myocardial infarction, and heart failure (Kachur et al., 2017). The most effective therapies at reversing CVD risk factors associated with obesity have been dietary changes with exercise, primarily through structured exercise programs (Kachur et al., 2017). The risk of heart disease continued to increases as BMI increases, doubling in overweight people to more than ten times in severely obese people compared with individuals with a healthy BMI (Dwivedi et al., 2020; Kivimaki et al., 2017). The PCPs are recommended to screen for other chronic diseases in overweight and obese patients to prevent developing a CVD (Kivimaki et al., 2017).

A cross-sectional study was evaluated by Pollack et al. (2020) using a national health and nutrition examination survey data from 2007 to 2016, 14,243 adults in the U.S, to determine the prevalence of obesity-related multi-morbidity and cardiovascular disease. An interview was administered in the participants' homes or at a mobile examination center. The researchers used questionnaires to collect the obesity-related risk of chronic diseases (ORCD), hypertension, T2DM, coronary heart disease, and stroke. Pollack et al. (2020) set an alpha level of 0.05 to determine statistical significance, and statistical analyses were performed using STATA/SE 11.2 (Pollack et al., 2020). Pollack et al. (2020) found that class III obesity was associated with an increased risk of coronary heart disease (HR 1.6, 95% CI 1.0–2.4) and stroke (HR 1.8, 95% CI 1.3–2.5). It was also found that individuals with one pre-existing condition had a four to seven-fold increased risk of coronary heart disease, and individuals with pre-existing hypertension or coronary heart disease had a four-fold increased risk of stroke (Pollack et al., 2020). This study's strength was the large sample size; the limitation was the self-reported data on ORCD diagnoses, which could be subject to recall bias. Another limitation was using cross-sectional data, which could not detect BMI changes throughout the study period. Intervention strategies to reduce cardiovascular disease included preventing overweight and obesity and detecting and managing hypertension and diabetes before the cardiovascular disease.

A cross-sectional study was conducted by Ryu et al. (2019) to examine the association between obesity and hypertension among American adults between 1999 and 2014. The authors used the National Health and Nutrition Examination Survey (NHANES) to determine whether the magnitude of the association between obesity and hypertension changed over the last 15-years among the total sample size of 38,993 adults. The NHANES was an ongoing survey conducted by the CDC using a representative sample of non-institutionalized U.S civilians (Ryu et al., 2019). Obesity was determined by assessing BMI, hypertension, and self-reported medication use (Ryu et al., 2019). Meta-regression was used to determine the relationship between the observed odds ratio effect sizes (obesity and hypertension) and the NHANES cycles (year) using a random-effects model. Across the years of 1999 to 2014, there was a significant positive linear trend ($p = .006$) in the association between overweight/obesity and hypertension. The researchers concluded that the association between overweight, obesity, and hypertension was becoming stronger over time (Ryu et al., 2019). The recommendation includes continuing surveillance of changes associated with obesity and hypertension to monitor how such changes may underlie chronic disease (Ryu et al., 2019).

Shrestha et al. (2021) used a qualitative study to explore 22 participants' knowledge of complications of obesity through focus group discussions. The 22 participants had BMI greater than 25 kg/m^2. Data were analyzed using the hybrid thematic analysis approach. The transcripts were analyzed and grouped text units using the Atlas.ti V.7. Musculoskeletal problems, such as difficulty sitting and walking, back pain, and pressure on the heel due to overweight were the predominant complications reported by participants. Many also reported high blood pressure, high cholesterol, and heart disease as complications. Participants' knowledge of complications was not only based on their experience but also on what they had seen in their family and community. The strength of the study includes in-depth views of overweight and obese patients on the complication of obesity. The study provided information on obesity and its perceived threat in a resource-poor setting. The study is limited to 22 participants residing in a suburban area; therefore, the study's findings may not be transferable to rural or urban areas. Nevertheless, the study has generated recommendations and possible strategies for obesity prevention in the vulnerable population.

Khan et al. (2018) used a prospective cohort to examine the association of BMI with CVD morbidity and mortality among 190 672 adults. The authors hypothesized that overweight or obesity would be associated with greater lifetime CVD risk compared with normal BMI. The individual-level data were pooled from adults aged 20 to 89. All participants were free of clinical CVD at baseline with available BMI index and CVD outcomes data. All statistical analyses were performed using SAS version 9.2, and Kaplan-Meier analysis was used to determine the lifetime risk. Khan et al. (2018) reported that the hazard ratios for the incident of CVD among middle-aged men and women for normal weight were (BMI of 18.5 to 24.9), 1.21 (95% CI, 1.14-1.28), and 1.32 (95% CI, 1.24-1.40), respectively, for overweight (BMI, 25.0-29.9), 1.67 (95% CI, 1.55-1.79) and 1.85 (95% CI, 1.72-1.99) for obesity (BMI, 30.0-39.9), and 3.14 (95% CI, 2.48-3.97) and 2.53 (95% CI, 2.20-2.91) for morbid obesity (BMI, ≥40.0). The lifetime risk for incidents of CVD was more significant in adults who were overweight and obese adults had an earlier onset of incident CVD and shorter overall survival compared with adults with normal BMI (Khan et al., 2018). The strengths include the 50 years duration of the study and the large sample size of adults free of CVD at baseline. The limitation of the study was the use of baseline BMI at index ages without accounting for the change in BMI across follow-up. The authors recommended the analysis of inception cohorts of people at the time of CVD diagnosis to detect if the finding will lead to risks of being overweight

Someya et al. (2018) conducted a cohort study of 636 Japanese male alumni of the physical education school to investigate the relationship between BMI at a young age and the future development of hypertension. The authors hypothesized that BMI at a young age was associated with hypertension later in life. The data were obtained from the physical examination at college-age and follow-up investigation between 2007 and 2011. The authors used standardized physical examination data of the alumni recorded when the participants were college students and data from medical examination of self-administered questionnaires at follow-up investigation to test the study hypothesis. The alumni were asked about their medical history whether they had ever been diagnosed with any disease, including hypertension, by a physician after graduation from college. Alumni were also asked about their current lifestyles, such as exercise, diet, and smoking habits. During the follow-up period, 120 men developed hypertension. Someya et al. (2018), found that the prevalence rates of hypertension for lowest to highest BMI categories were 9.4%, 14.6%, 16.1%, 17.5%, 30.3%, and 29.3%, respectively ($p<0.001$ for trend), and their hazard ratios were 1.00 (reference), 1.80 (95%CI: 0.65–4.94), 2.17 (0.83–5.64), 2.29 (0.89–5.92), 3.60 (1.37–9.47) and 4.72 (1.78–12.48), respectively (p<0.001 for trend). The authors concluded that slightly increased BMI at a young age was a significant risk factor for future hypertension in Japanese men (Someya et al., 2018). There were several limitations to the study. First, the participants were not representative of all Japanese men, and female alumni were omitted. Second, self-selection bias could have occurred because the participants who answered the follow-up questionnaires might have been those who were the healthiest. Alumni without data of either the physical examination while at college or follow-up questionnaire were excluded. These exclusions limited the generalization of the results. Third, recall bias was possible because the questionnaire was cross-sectional, and participants needed to recall their medical history. The inclusion of female and male participants from several schools was recommended for future studies.

In summary, awareness and knowledge of obesity-related risks such as CVD are important in managing overweight and obesity in primary settings. Many researchers examined the association between obesity and CVD, and all reported that obesity was a chronic health condition and had a higher risk factor for developing CVD (Khan et al., 2018; Pollack et al., 2020; Ryu et al., 2019; Shrestha et al., 2021; Someya et al., 2018). Intervention strategies to reduce obesity-related risk must start from preventing overweight and obesity and detecting and managing an early diagnosis of chronic diseases before the onset of cardiovascular disease.

Overweight and Obesity Intervention

Obesity specialists developed multiple treatment guidelines to provide guidance and support to PCPs diagnosing and managing overweight and obesity. Management of adults with overweight and obesity involved clinical guidelines based on evidence-based practice to guide PCPs improved patients' health outcomes (Dols et al., 2017; Mackey & Bassendowski, 2017). Evidence-based practice was a problem-solving approach used in clinical decision-making within a health care organization that integrated the best available scientific evidence for the application of an intervention (Fineout-Overholt, 2019). The PCPs played a significant role in guiding patients to incorporate healthy eating and physical activity habits into a routine visit. Approaches to weight loss were lifestyle modification, physical activity, pharmacotherapy, and surgical intervention (Gibbs et al., 2017; Taylor, 2020); however, pharmacotherapy and surgery were not part of interventions for this project.

American Heart Association, American College of Cardiology, and The Obesity Society guidelines. In 2014, a panel representing experts from the AHA, ACC, and TOS, among other stakeholders, developed a set of guidelines and recommendations for PCPs to manage overweight and obesity in adults (Jensen et al., 2014). The AHA, ACC, and TOS guidelines were based on high-quality randomized trials, meta-analyses, and observational studies by a panel of experts on each subject (Jensen et al., 2014). The overall objective of these guidelines was to assess obesity-related risk and reduce the onset of the disease by encouraging people who are at risk to engage in lifestyle modifications. The guidelines were directed toward PCP (doctors, APNs, and PAs) to help support overweight and obesity management in primary care practice (Jensen et al., 2014). The AHA, ACC, and TOS guidelines recommended a “grade A” level of confidence for BMI. The 2014 AHA, ACC, and TOS guidelines recommend using a BMI range from 25 to 29.9 kg/m2 to classify overweight and a BMI cut-off point of 30 kg/m2 and higher to classify obesity in adult individuals with increased CVD risk. BMI presents limitations in predicting the body fat association with health risk individually (Jensen et al., 2014). Another limitation of BMI is that when lifestyle interventions are applied, this measurement is not an accurate indicator of an improved health outcome, sometimes causing disappointment and diet and exercise regimens abandonment.

Wadden et al. (2020) used AHA, ACC, and TOS guidelines for managing overweight and obesity in adults as a framework to explore the principal components of comprehensive lifestyle modification, which include diet, physical activity, and behavior therapy. The guideline has recommended that PCPs screen all adults for obesity and provide those affected intensive, multicomponent lifestyle interventions. The AHA, ACC, and TOS guidelines recommended for individuals to lose weight; the participation must include six months in high-intensity programs that provide 14 or more counseling sessions with a trained interventionist on a low-calorie diet and increase in physical activity. According to Wadden et al. (2020), when provided face-to-face individual or group treatment, participants lose up to 8 kg (8% of weight) in 6 months and experience improvements in cardiovascular disease risk factors and quality of life. High levels of physical activity, frequent monitoring of body weight, and consumption of a reduced-calorie diet are associated with long-term weight loss (Wadden et al., 2020). The strength of the study is the six-month duration of interventions. The researchers recommended using this intervention with digitally delivered programs because it will lower costs, expand treatment reach, and improve monitoring of food intake, activity, and weight. Ultimately, to improve long-term weight management, individual lifestyle modification must be joined with collective and institutional efforts to improve the nation's eating and physical activity.

Reis et al. (2018) examined the quality of clinical guidelines for managing adult overweight and obesity using the appraisal of guidelines for research and evaluation (AGREE). The researchers included the following criteria: (1) clinical guidelines for overweight and obesity, (2) treatment recommendations for adults, and (3) involvement of a government agency and state-level of health professionals. Twenty-three guidelines were identified from seventeen countries. The consistency between the scoring processes points to the AGREE II's reliability as a quality assessment instrument (Reis et al., 2018). The authors indicated that the scope of practice and presentation had the highest score, while applicability and stakeholder involvement had the lowest score. The limitation of using the AGREE II instrument was a lack of inclusion of the monitoring process and the use of the PICOT question, which was also recommended by the authors (Reis et al., 2018).

Alagoz et al. (2018) conducted a randomized controlled trial systematic review comprised of 21 studies in nine countries, with 13 studies in the United States. Most of the studies focused on clinical guidelines related to chronic health conditions, including obesity. The strategies investigated in the studies included clinical guidelines, provision of educational materials, practice facilitation, and system support. The studies varied regarding the type and number of interventions. Nine of the studies measured the effects of an intervention with two components, while others evaluated the impact of interventions with three or more components. Clinical guidelines were used as a multi-faceted intervention in 16 trials, and 11 of the trials used practice facilitation as an intervention. Thirteen of the 21 studies reported statistically significant improvement ($p < .05$) in their primary outcome utilizing clinical guidelines. Four studies described mixed results: a substantial increase in some outcomes with no improvement in others. Five of the six studies that showed no improvement in outcomes using clinical guidelines had no follow-up. Some reasons identified for the lack of effect between the control and experimental group include lack of follow-up. Alagoz et al. (2018) support clinical guidelines, especially as components in a multi-faceted intervention. Alagoz et al. (2018) indicate clinical guidelines can increase the uptake and care in chronic disease management. Alagoz et al. (2018) indicate the continual, regular follow-up and presence of the facilitator in managing chronic diseases. Alagoz et al. (2018) suggested providing printed educational materials, an electronic support system, in-person education, and regular, frequent follow-up is needed to promote change.

Lopez (2016) used a cross-sectional study to assess adult 753 participants' weight and blood pressure changes in a weight treatment program. The AHA/ACC/TOS guidelines were used as a reference to evaluate weight and blood pressure changes between pre-and post-intervention. The specific aims of the study were. 1) to identify participants who upon enrollment met the AHA, ACC, and TOS Guideline cut-off points for overweight and obesity; 2) to identify participants who, in addition to meeting the overweight and obesity criteria, 3) to determine the proportion of female and male participants who achieved 3, 5 and 10 percent weight reduction. It is hypothesized that adults eligible to lose weight among participants, as established by the AHA, ACC, and TOS guidelines for managing overweight and obesity in adults. A secondary hypothesis is that among the selected sample of participating adults who completed the intervention and reached or exceed the weight loss reduction of 5% will have a clinically meaningful outcome in blood pressure measurements. The IBM SPSS statistic software (SPSS-version 22) was used for analysis. The median weight loss of 1.31±3.3 kg was statistically significant (p=0.001), representing a 0.5±1.29 kg/m2 (p=0.001) decrease in overall BMI measurements. A total of 28% of the 285 selected participants who completed the PLMM achieved a bodyweight loss of 3% or more, which will produce clinically meaningful health benefits according to the AHA, ACC, and TOS guidelines. Lopez (2016) recommended that an individualized diet component and increased intervention time to 6 months or more could further improve the health benefits.

In summary, the PCPs are positioned to treat patients with overweight and obesity, influencing and impacting the course of the disease using clinical practice guidelines. Finding the best evidence to help guide the management of overweight and obesity using evidence-based guidelines was critical to develop an intervention to improve the use of the AHA, ACC, and TOS guidelines. All studies that included clinical guidelines reported significant effects in one or more outcomes (Alagoz et al., 2018; Lopez, 2016; Wadden et al., 2020). One study that examined the quality of clinical guidelines for managing adult overweight noted consistency and reliability in the quality of 23 clinical guidelines identified. The authors indicated that the scope of practice and presentation had the highest score, while applicability had the lowest score (Reis et al., 2018).

The American Association of Clinical Endocrinologists and the American College of Endocrinology (AACE-ACE). The AACE-ACE created a chronic care model, advanced diagnostic framework, clinical practice guidelines, and clinical practice algorithm for the comprehensive management of obesity. The guideline emphasizes lifestyle modification in promoting overall health, not only as of the first algorithmic step but also as the central, pervasive action (Mechanick et al., 2017).

Turner et al. (2018) used a qualitative method to examine 1,506 primary care providers' (medical doctors, nurse practitioners, and obstetrics-gynecology) knowledge of evidence-based guidelines for overweight and obesity management. The investigator included only those who practice in the primary care settings and practice for at least three years. It is essential to know that participants received an honorarium of $21 to $90 upon completing the survey. Self-reported weight and height were used to calculate each participant's BMI. The data were collected using DocStyloes. X^2 test, odds ratios, and generalized linear models were used to assess differences in provider responses. Turner et al. (2018) found that 16% of participants indicated that overweight and obesity intervention should be provided twice a month for six months. Only 15% of participants identified BMI greater than 27 kg/m^2 with obesity commodities that should be considered for pharmacotherapy (Turner et al., 2018). The results of the study suggest that respondents lack knowledge of obesity treatment guidelines. The study did not include physician assistants; therefore, it limits generalization to all health care practitioners. The overall finding that healthcare professionals care for obese patients is inconsistent with the evidence-based recommendation, therefore recommended training programs.

Kovacs et al. (2018) explored the effectiveness of various implementation strategies in clinical guidelines in systematic review and meta-analysis. This high-quality, Grade A review included 36 studies. A harvest plot was completed with the 36 studies, and a forest plot was completed with 21 of the studies. Some studies tested a single intervention, while others tested a multi-faceted intervention that included two or more interventions. According to this review, a single diverse intervention such as n such as "audit, reminder, lifestyle modification, motivational interviewing, or patient-mediated had the greatest effect with 73% of outcome indicators being effective; 0.48 [0.38, 0.58]" for all outcomes except counseling (Kovacs et al., 2018, p. 1149). Lifestyle interventions had 65% of indicators being effective 0.11 [0.01, 0.20] (Kovacs et al., 2018). The least effective method of implementation was the passive distribution of materials. Educational outreach plus audit and feedback resulted in a decrease in either intervention alone (38% of the indicators showing any effect). Other combinations did not dramatically decrease but were not as effective as the single method. The authors recommend lifestyle modification and interactive educational outreach as opposed to passive didactic sessions. While Kovacs et al. (2018) do not indicate improved outcomes with a multi-faceted approach, each component of the multi-faceted intervention (low-calorie diet and physical activity) for this project does demonstrate a positive effect.

The evidence summary by Gomersall (2017) evaluates the role of healthcare teams and guideline dissemination. This evidence summary examined the role of healthcare teams in guideline dissemination. The overview also reviewed the effect of printed educational materials (PEM), lifestyle modification, and feedback. PEMs, when used as a single intervention and compared to no intervention, had a small but beneficial outcome on professional practice (Gomersall, 2017). Lifestyle modification and feedback had small improvements in practice. Evidence suggests that multiple approaches should be considered when implementing guidelines, including PEM, lifestyle modification, and feedback. It also stresses the importance that all team members understand the guidelines (Gomersall, 2017). Gomersall (2017) demonstrates the need for a multi-faceted approach to guideline dissemination. Gomersall (2017) noted that reminders showed a small improvement in professional practice, which was also noted with lifestyle modification.

In summary, clinical practice guidelines represent the most important evidence-based decision support tool, and several strategies have been applied to improve their implementation in primary care settings. Studies evaluate the effect of clinical intervention methods on the guideline adherence of PCPs. The three studies covering interventions using multiple and single interventions based on clinical guidelines did not find a similar result. One study found that single interventions were the most effective, and distribution of materials was the least effective management of overweight and obesity (Kovacs et al., 2018). Another study found that multiple interventions were more effective than a single intervention (Gomersall, 2017). The result of another revealed that PCPs lack knowledge of obesity management guidelines, therefore, education. The study did not include physician assistants; consequently, it limits generalization to all health care practitioners. The overall finding that healthcare professionals care for obese patients is inconsistent with the evidence-based recommendation, therefore recommended training programs.

Obesity Medicine Association. The OMA was published with a comprehensive algorithm that incorporated individualized strategies that enabled PCPs to counsel patients for dieting, exercising, behavioral counseling, pharmacological management, and when to consult a specialist (Bays et al., 2019). The OMA guidelines aimed to improve overweight and obesity management and developed care standards regarding at-risk patients with other chronic conditions (Bays et al., 2019).

Disser (2019) used a retrospective study to determine if evidence-based practice guidelines would increase the rate of diagnosis and treatment of patients with overweight and obesity in primary care. The participants were 13 advanced practice registered nurses. Descriptive statistics were used to compare data obtained retrospectively through a 2-week chart review pre- and post-intervention. There were no statistically significant differences between the two groups. Utilizing one-tailed z-scores, statistical significance was found in two of the four primary outcomes. There was an increase in diagnoses after the evidence-based practice guidelines intervention in patients with overweight ($z = -1.8$, $p = .04$). There was also an increase in documented treatment post-intervention in patients with obesity ($z = -2.23$, $p = .01$). The strength of this study is the use of multiple sites (urban, suburban, and rural), which increased the generalizability of the findings. The study had several limitations, most notably, the sample size and selection. As noted, 13 APRNs were self-selected, which creates bias. The size of the sample is too small to draw any real conclusions.

Slade (2018) used a quantitative study to examine the effects of utilizing evidence-based practice guidelines on weight loss implementation. This evidence summary looked at several studies which examined several interventions. The recommendations for this evidence summary were synthesized from two systematic reviews, a before and after study (N=19), an RCT (N=4530), a pilot RCT (N=35), a retrospective cohort with a time-series analysis, and a non-RCT (N=101). The summary recommends multiple interventions with a Grade A recommendation either alone or in combination with other strategies. The evidence shows a small but consistent effect, especially regarding lifestyle intervention prescribing behaviors. The characteristics of the practitioners, aspects of targeted behavior, and the context of the intervention should be considered before developing the intervention (Slade, 2018). This evidence summary by Slade (2018) provides evidence on the positive effect of lifestyle intervention using evidence-based guidelines. Although the results were mixed for complex behaviors, some studies reported a significant impact. One pilot study (N=35) reported 58% of general practitioners in the experimental arm changed the management of patients with obesity and reported an increase in their knowledge and confidence after the intervention (Slade, 2018).

Egger et al. (2017) performed a quasi-experimental, longitudinal study to determine the effects of organizational and evidence-based practice interventions on adherence to clinical practice guidelines in Kenya. The authors used the regular staff as the intervention group and the locum staff as the control group. The intervention consisted of online learning modules on the use of evidenced-based practice guidelines. Guideline adherence at baseline was 41.4% for the regular staff and 26.5% for the locum staff. At the end of the trial, the regular staff increased to 77.1%, and the locum staff decreased to 21.8%. This study demonstrates the effects of interventions to improve adherence to guidelines (Egger et al., 2017). Although the research was done in a low-resource setting, many of the clinics in the Medical Group are in rural underserved areas with limited resource availability. Even in resource-rich regions, as reimbursement rates decrease, low-cost implementation strategies become essential in all locations. The outcomes support the use of evidence-based practice intervention on the guideline uptake. The interventions used in this quasi-experiment provide substantial evidence to support the utilization of this EBP project.

In summary, clinical guidelines are routinely incorporated into evidence-based practice to help improve health outcomes. While there are many ways to implement knowledge, the evidence consistently shows measurable improvement in practice utilizing evidence-based practice guidelines (Disser, 2019; Eggar et al., 2018; Slade, 2018). Determining and translating the evidence-based strategies to guide the dissemination of evidence-based clinical practice guidelines and knowledge was the focus of the literature review and synthesis

Diet and Physical Activity. Successful overweight and obesity management required integrating a low-calorie diet and physical activity. Once a patient has decided to lose weight, assessing weight or obesity begins with evaluating the patient's risk, goals, and recommendations for treatment goals (Bays et al., 2019; Chan et al., 2017).

Hall and Guo (2017) used a correlational design to compare the three conceptual models of energy balance regulation. The human body's implications with the dynamics of carbohydrate, fat, and protein on energy balance, body weight, and composition were evaluated Hall & Guo, 2017). Thirty-two studies were reviewed to answer whether all diet calories were created equal regarding the effects of carbohydrate, fat, and protein on energy balance, body weight, and composition. According to Hall and Guo (2017), there was a weight loss plateau after six months with no further loss, despite continued intervention. Hall and Guo (2017) found that after the intervention stopped, the energy intake increased above the baseline. The pooled weighted mean differences across the studies demonstrated small differences in daily energy expenditure (26 kcal/d, $p< 0.0001$) and body fat change (16 kcal/d $p < 0.0001$), favoring low-calorie diets (Hall & Guo, 2017).

Bear et al. (2020) used a cluster-randomized trial l to evaluate the effect of an online weight management program integrated with population health management on weight change. Participants included 840 overweight and obese with hypertension or T2DM between ages 20 to 70 with BMI body 27kg/m2 and < 40 kg/m2 from 15 practices. Participants were assigned to the usual care group (n=326) that received general information about weight management, the online-only group (n = 216)) which included meal plans, physical activity, and progress reporting features, and the combined intervention group (n = 298) receiving additional outreach and support. The primary outcome was weight change at 12 months, and weight change at 18 months was a secondary outcome. The result indicated there was a significant difference in weight change at 12 months by the group with a mean weight change of –1.2 kg (95% CI, –2.1 to –0.3 kg) in the usual care group, –1.9 kg (95% CI, –2.6 to –1.1 kg) in the online program only group, and –3.1 kg (95% CI, –3.7 to –2.5 kg) in the combined intervention group ($P < .001$). The result indicated that a combination of dietary counseling and physical activity improves weight loss. Bear et al. (2020) recommended further research to understand the generalizability and durability of the findings.

A quantitative study was used by Whelam et al. (2017) to examine the effectiveness of evidence-based lifestyle intervention weight management targeting physical activity, healthy eating, and weight loss services in the outpatient clinic. A primary health care organization provided a telephone-delivered healthy lifestyle and weight loss program. The investigators used a single-group, repeated measures design; outcomes were assessed at six months (mid-program; $n = 166$) and 12-month (end of the program; n = 88) using paired analyses (Whelam et al., 2017). The sixty-three percent of participants referred for lifestyle counseling was significantly increased over time (4.4%-50%), P< 0.001; Whelan et al., 2017). The study demonstrated a statistically significant improvement between baseline and end of the program for weight [mean change (SE) -5.4 (7.0) kg] and waist circumference [-4.8 (9.7) cm], underpinned by significant physical activity and dietary change (Whelam et al., 2017).

Barghi et al. (2017) used a semi-experimental pretest-posttest design with the control group. The effectiveness of an independent variable (lifestyle modification) was investigated on dependent variables of weight management, body image, and sexual self-esteem. Thirty adult women between ages 18 and 38 with a BMI of 30 kg/m^2 or greater participated in the study. The participants were randomly assigned to the training intervention group based on lifestyle modification [experimental group] and control group. The pretest was administered to both groups. The experimental group was subjected to lifestyle modification training, and the control group did not receive any intervention. The treatment sessions consisted of 12 sessions of 90 minutes performed collectively and once a week. Post-tests were administered to both groups, and then the data were analyzed by MANCOVA. Lifestyle modification had a significant effect on multidimensional self-body relations (28, 1) =243.337, p<0.001, weight efficacy lifestyle (28, 1) =328.860, p<0.001, and sexual self-esteem) (28.1) =284.228, p<0.001 was significant. The finding indicates an increase in multi-dimensional self-body relations, weight efficacy lifestyle, and self-esteem. In the experimental group, compare the control group. The strength of the study was the use of the experimental method. The limitation of the study includes the convenience sampling method, small sample size, and self-reporting tools. Barghi et al. (2017) suggested more controlled studies on this treatment's effectiveness for other variables such as mental health in overweight women.

In summary, weight-loss interventions utilizing low calorie and physical activity is the first step in weight loss management. The literature review findings suggested some crucial and challenging factors in weight-loss intervention effectiveness, such as increased physical activity and dietary changes. The most significant weight loss participants reported were consuming a low-calorie diet, more vegetables, fruit, and were more likely to eat low-fat food (Barghi et al., 2017; Bear et al., 2020; Whelam et al., 2017). Documentation of exercise habits and recommendations for those not attaining 150 minutes per week promoted compliance were found to gain more weight (Hall & Guo, 2017). This project involved counseling overweight and obese patients on low-calorie diets of their choice and walking for 150 minutes or more per week. There was no single effective intervention for weight loss management. All studies reported a combination of diet and physical activity for effective weight loss intervention.

Summary

The literature review covered obesity-related risk and complication, overweight, and obesity intervention. The TGA and HBM were models used to implement this direct practice improvement project. These frameworks provided a foundation for understanding weight loss and obesity risk knowledge and developing an effective intervention to improve clinical outcomes at the project site. The purpose of this quantitative quasi-experimental quality improvement project was to determine if the implementation of the American Heart Association, American College of Cardiology, and The Obesity Society (AHA/ACC/TOS) *Guidelines for the Management of*

Overweight and Obesity in Adults would impact weight, body mass index (BMI), and obesity risk knowledge among adults with BMI greater than 25 kg/m^2. The project was completed over four weeks in a primary care clinic in central California. This literature review guided the process of consistently implementing evidence-based interventions for overweight and obesity management in the primary care setting.

The literature review indicated a need to prevent and treat the overweight and obesity epidemic. Management of overweight and obese patients involved using evidence-based clinical guidelines to improve patients' health outcomes (Bays et al., 2019; Jensen et al., 2014; Mechanick et al., 2017). The strength of the clinical guidelines was the rigorous and comprehensive literature review. Weight loss was recommended for all overweight or obese patients regardless of comorbid conditions. After synthesizing the literature on obesity risk and complication, the researchers found that obese individuals had low obesity risk knowledge and misperceived their body weight as obese. The findings from the literature review also revealed that the higher the BMI, the more likely the individuals would develop cancers, T2DM, or CVD. Therefore, there was a need to continue to improve counseling regarding the risks of being overweight or obese.

Several weight management guidelines were mainly related to lifestyle modifications. A project was needed to examine the effect of clinical guidelines, specifically from AHA, ACC, and TOS, to manage overweight and obesity in the primary care setting. The literature review found a single intervention such as dietary, physical activity, medication, or behavior therapy proved successful without incorporating other interventions, suggesting a gap in practice. This project manager found from this literature review that the treatment must be a combination of interventions to achieve weight loss outcomes. There was an opportunity for the project to move forward with translating the evidence-based AHA, ACC, and TOS guidelines into practice with the hope of improving weight loss outcomes in the primary care setting. The intervention's focus was individualized while adhering to the recommendation by evidenced-based guidelines, as demonstrated by the literature review (Barghi et al., 2017; Bear et al., 2020; Wadden et al., 2020).

Through this direct practice improvement project, the proposal was planned for implementing evidence-based interventions established by the AHA, ACC, and TOS guidelines to manage overweight and obesity among adult patients in the primary care setting. APNs were prepared to take full responsibility in selecting appropriate interventions in managing overweight and obesity in a primary care setting, as noted in the theme of the overweight and obesity intervention (Disser, 2019; Lopez, 2016; Reis et al., 2018; Wadden et al., 2020). The TGA and HBM were selected as the most appropriate theoretical frameworks to accomplish the project. The theories provided an understanding of health-promoting behaviors (increased weight loss as evidenced by BMI; improved knowledge of obesity-related risk) and assisted in developing appropriate and effective interventions at the project site.

The problem identified at the project site was that the APNs did not have standardized clinical guidelines for managing overweight and obesity. Therefore, it was not known if AHA, ACC, and TOS implementation would improve weight loss outcomes and increase obesity risk knowledge. The population selected for chart audit was adult patients between 18 to 64 years with BMI 26kg/m^2 or higher, seen by APNs during the project implementation. The project was conducted at a primary care setting located in central California. A quantitative quasi-experimental with a pre-intervention and post-intervention was the methodology used for the project. The independent variable was the AHA, ACC, and TOS guidelines, and the dependent variables were weight, BMI, and obesity risk knowledge. The literature supported using the evidence-based AHA, ACC, and TOS guidelines for managing overweight and obesity in the primary care setting. There was a gap in the literature concerning overweight and obesity management using evidence-based clinical guidelines, and the project had addressed the gap. Chapter 3 presents the project methodology, design, sample selection, instrumentation of the quantitative project, validity, reliability, data collection, and data analysis procedures. Ethical considerations and project limitations are also discussed in Chapter 3.

Chapter 3: Methodology

This quantitative quality improvement project seeks to answer whether utilizing AHA, ACC, and TOS guidelines by APRNs in a primary care setting would improve weight loss and obesity risk knowledge among overweight and obesity. The purpose of this quantitative quasi-experimental quality improvement project was to determine if the implementation of the American Heart Association, American College of Cardiology, and The Obesity Society (AHA/ACC/TOS) *Guidelines for the Management of Overweight and Obesity in Adults* would impact weight, body mass index (BMI), and obesity risk knowledge among adults with BMI greater than 25 kg/m^2. The project was completed over four weeks in a primary care clinic in central California. The project focused on reducing weight and BMI and increased obesity risk knowledge among patients who received intervention provided by APNs using AHA, ACC, and TOS guidelines as a reference. Despite the availability of different evidence-based clinical guidelines for managing overweight and obesity, little was known if implementing the AHA, ACC, and TOS guidelines in a primary care setting would improve weight loss outcomes (change in weight, BMI) and obesity risk knowledge.

Chapter 3 elaborates on the quantitative methodology and quasi-experimental design of the project. The population and sample selection process will also be discussed. Data collection instruments, as well as data collection procedures and data analysis procedures, will be addressed. The validity and reliability of the tools are reviewed. Additionally, topics discussed in Chapter 3 also include potential biases, ethical considerations, limitations, and a summary.

Statement of the Problem

It was not known if or to what degree the implementation of the American Heart Association, American College of Cardiology, and The Obesity Society (AHA/ACC/TOS) *Guidelines for the Management of Overweight and Obesity in Adults* would impact weight, body mass index (BMI), and obesity risk knowledge among adults with BMI greater than 25 kg/m2. Patients with obesity and overweight were often addressed during the office visits at the project site; however, patients were given very few ongoing weight management guidelines. This direct practice improvement project contributed to solving overweight and obesity by providing an evidence-based practice, AHA, ACC, and TOS, to positively impact weight reduction and improve obesity risk knowledge in adult patients seen at the participating practice.

The problem associated with managing overweight and obesity is not simply an issue of low self-control concerning foods or a lack of motivation to move; instead, it is a chronic disease that requires routine intervention (Bays et al., 2019; Jensen et al., 2014. Even though clinical practice guidelines are available, the under-treatment of overweight and obesity in primary care persists (Hayes et al., 2017). Overweight and obesity guidelines are available for PCPs, including APNs, for review, complete with the chief recommendation to assess obesity as part of routine screening and wellness visits, yet, PCPs fail to follow through consistently (Huff et al., 2020).

Clinical Question

The clinical question for this project was: To what degree did the implementation of Jensen's Guideline for the Management of Overweight and Obesity in Adults from the AHA, ACC, and TOS impact weight, BMI, and obesity risk knowledge when compared to current practice among adults with BMI greater than 25 kg/m^2 in a primary care clinic in central California? Implementing the AHA, ACC, and TOS guidelines would help APNs focus on preventing and managing overweight and obesity at the project site located in central California. This project's independent variable was the AHA, ACC, and TOS guidelines, evidence-based clinical guidelines for managing overweight and obesity in primary care settings. The dependent variable was the patient outcomes (reduction in weight, BMI, and an increase in obesity risk knowledge). The weight was measured with the same scale by the same MA pre-intervention and post-interception. Obesity risk knowledge was measured using the ORK-10 questionnaire.

The project's focus was implementing the AHA, ACC, and TOS guidelines published in 2014 for managing overweight and obesity in primary care settings (Jensen et al., 2014). APNs at the project site implemented the AHA, ACC, and TOS guidelines to identify patients who needed interventions to prevent obesity-related diseases. The primary outcome measure was to reduce weight and BMI and assess the participant's knowledge of obesity risk.

Project Methodology

A quantitative research methodology was used for the project due to its ability to provide numerical data regarding the relationship between variables (AHA, ACC, and TOS guidelines and patient outcomes of weight, BMI, and obesity risk knowledge). The rationale for choosing a quantitative method was implementing an evidence-based AHA, ACC, and TOS guideline for improvement and analyzing the data before and after the intervention.

The qualitative method is a subjective methodology wherein the investigator is the primary instrument for data collection compared to quantitative instruments such as databases and control groups used for data collection. In nursing doctoral projects, qualitative methods are also valuable to data collection when implementing intervention and not considering its outcomes. Experiences, configurations in an individual's world, and life occurrences are the outcomes the qualitative project manager evaluates. These outcomes indicate the qualitative learner is interested in the process, interpretation, and awareness acquired from the qualitative data. Examples of qualitative design methods are subjective sources such as polls, questionnaires, and interviews. In qualitative methods, the learner is the primary instrument for data collection compared to quantitative instruments such as databases and control groups used for data collection. The basic difference between quantitative and qualitative methods is described using philosophical bases. Quantitative methods are based on positivism principles such as objective world reality, whereas qualitative methods use phenomena to explore humans' responses and how society is influenced (Cathala & Moorley, 2019).

Quantitative methods allow the project manager to examine a theory using a highly structured design method and present sound outcomes validated by science. Consideration for validity, reliability, and applicability was taken into consideration with a quantitative methodology. This project may be the only practical method of assessing an intervention's impact due to the pre-intervention and post-intervention questionnaires (Cathala & Moorley, 2019). Therefore, this quantitative methodology was the appropriate methodology to use for the pre and post-intervention of the AHA, ACC, and TOS guidelines. According to Apuke (2017), a quantitative method involves utilizing and analyzing numerical data using specific statistical techniques to answer questions like who, how much, what, where, when, how many, and how. The quantitative study also describes the methods of explaining an issue through gathering data in numerical form (Apuke, 2017). The project aimed to examine if AHA, ACC, and TOS guidelines would affect weight, BMI, and obesity risk knowledge in central California. The association exists between two variables when the change in one variable influences another variable being studied (Cathala & Moorley, 2019). Causal is defined as the proof that the adjustment in the independent variable (AHA, ACC, and TOS guidelines) leads to a change in the dependent variable (weight, BMI, and obesity risk knowledge).

Project Design

The rationale for selecting a quasi-experimental design was implementing an evidence-based intervention to improve and analyze the data before and after the intervention using descriptive statistics (Maciejewski, 2020). A quasi-experimental design was the best approach for the project because the plan was viewed as an intervention in which treatment was being evaluated for how well it achieved its objectives, as measured by pre-intervention and post-intervention. Two variables were reviewed for causation (Maciejewski, 2020). The design allowed manipulation of the independent variable to define the intervention's causal effect on the dependent variables to answer the clinical questions without randomization (Maciejewski, 2020; Miller et al., 2020). The design provided the opportunity to use descriptive statistics to compare two points in time: baseline and following the intervention for the project question (Maciejewski, 2020). As a result of the intervention, any change in characteristics measured was likely attributable to implementing the AHA, ACC, and TOS guidelines.

The project collected data from patients' paper charts using pre and post-intervention chart review to identify if the independent variable (AHA, ACC, and TOS) would impact dependent variables (change in weight, BMI, and obesity risk knowledge). APNs implemented the AHA, ACC, and TOS guidelines to determine how it would benefit overweight and obese patients' outcomes (the dependent variable). Two different data collection tools were used: the AHRQ Tool 2 Chart Audit Form to collect demographics and tracking weight management. The ORK-10 established obesity risk knowledge at baseline and post-intervention through a paper chart audit for the quantitative project. The chart reviews helped establish the impact of AHA, ACC, and TOS guidelines on patient outcomes and the APNs' ability to apply evidence-based interventions to improve overweight and obesity management at the project site. The paired sample *t*-test was performed using the Statistical Package for the Social Sciences (SPSS) software that compared patient outcomes before and after the AHA, ACC, and TOS implementation.

Population and Sample Selection

This direct practice improvement project was implemented in a primary care clinic setting in California's central region. In the general overweight and obesity population, approximately 40% are classified as obese in central California (Elflein, 2020). The project site represents an example of high risk for overweight and obesity, with about 1200 patients who receive primary care services. The project site was a growing healthcare system that provided comprehensive primary care to the participant pool derived from patients who received care at the project site.

The clinic was staffed by a medical doctor, three APNs, one office manager, two billers, and five medical assistants. The APNs in this primary care setting managed approximately 30-40 patients per day, nearly all of whom lived in the city where the project site was located. The clinic also served as urgent care for walk-ins; however, since the Coronavirus pandemic, the operating hours changed from 8 am to 8 pm to 10 am to 6 pm for three days weekly for an onsite visit and two days for a telemedicine visit. Coronaviruses are related viruses that cause respiratory tract infections to spread through droplets released into the air when infected persons cough or sneezes (Liu & Liu, 2020). The Coronavirus droplets do not travel more than a few feet; therefore, physical distancing effectively prevents the disease's spread (Liu & Liu, 2020). To prevent the spread of Coronavirus at the project site, the number of patients seen daily by each APN decreased from 35 to 15-20.

Criteria for inclusion to the project included: (a) the patient was between age 18 and 64; (b) the patient had BMI >25 kg/m^2; (c) the patient was a resident of central California; and (d) the patient was receiving primary care services at the project site project. Exclusions from the participation included patients who were seen for urgent care needs. The sample size required for this project was determined with a G* power statistical analysis. An A Priori power analysis was done using the following measurements: power =.80, alpha = .05, and effect size = .25. The results indicated that a minimum sample size of 27 patients would be needed to achieve a power level of 0.80 for this project. The participant sample included a sample of 28 overweight and obese patients between 18 and 64 years of age with a BMI of 25 kg/m^2 or greater. The sample size of 28 participants at the project site was used to determine if evidence-based AHA,

ACC, and TOS guidelines among overweight and obese patients impacted outcomes of weight, BMI, and obesity risk knowledge compared to their baseline data.

The reason for using a sample size of 28 participants was to help expand the variety of possible data for the analysis. Using this preset sample allowed selecting participants by predetermined criteria (Maciejewski, 2020). The comparison group for this project was the same participating patients. The project compared the pre-intervention data with the post-intervention data on the same group on a continuous variable. Descriptive statistics and a paired *t*-test were used to analyze a sample size of 28 patient charts by the project manager after four weeks of implementing AHA, ACC, and TOS guidelines by APNs. The data values were matched, which indicated that the paired *t*-test would be the most appropriate analysis (Anand, 2020). A paired *t*-test was conducted to compare the mean value of weight loss, BMI, and obesity risk knowledge at pre-intervention and post-intervention and addressed the clinical question by evaluating the impact of implementing the guidelines on patient weight, BMI, and obesity risk knowledge. During the regular office appointment with the APNs, all patients identified as overweight or obese by MA were treated by APNs using the AHA, ACC, and TOS guidelines as a reference.

Instrumentation and Sources of Data

The instrumentation and data source consisted of direct measurement in the project location of each participant at the beginning and end of the project. Each instrument used for the project was discussed separately below. Some of the instruments were evidence of reliability and validity, and most were available at no cost. The instruments were used for screening, diagnosis, management, or tracking of the treatment outcomes.

Obesity Risk Knowledge-10 (ORK-10)

Swift et al. (2006) developed the ORK-10 to evaluate the obesity risk knowledge of obese patients. The ORK-10 was a standardized and statistically significant predictor for obesity-risk knowledge utilizing a ten-question true or false answer assessment where one (1) point was given for each correct answer related to obesity-related risks. If the participant was unsure of a solution, they were given the option to select 'Do Not Know;' this was to help decrease the distorting effects of guessing. Swift et al. (2006) stated that the ORK-10 could effectively evaluate a person's health information related to obesity risk. The ORK-10 was used to assess the participants' knowledge of obesity-risk knowledge pre/post-intervention. APNs administered the questionnaires for those who met the inclusion criteria as BMI of 30 kg/m^2 or greater.

AHRQ Tool 2 Chart Audit Form

Tool 2 was developed by Agency for Healthcare Research and Quality (AHRQ) in 2014 for primary care practices to manage overweight and obesity (McGinnis et al., 2014). The AHRQ Tool 2 was used as a tracking tool for chart review to screen and manage overweight and obese patients (McGinnis et al., 2014). The AHRQ Tool 2 provides detailed step-by-step instructions for chart audit, including patient demographics, date of birth, gender, medical history, weight management intervention provided, and weight management tracking (height, weight, BMI, diet, exercise discussed, and weight management referral). For this project, weight management referral was not needed because APNs' adherence was not evaluated due to time constraints.

AHA, ACC, and TOS Clinical Guidelines

The AHA, ACC, and TOS guidelines were established and developed by health professionals for weight management in the primary care setting (Jensen et al., 2014). The AHA, ACC, and TOS guidelines were developed through an extensive literature review and evidence from rigorous research (Jensen et al., 2014). The AHA, ACC, and TOS guidelines were evidence-based to guide the PCPs' use as a reference in managing overweight and obese patients in the primary care setting. Evidence-based practice had been recognized as the key to improving healthcare quality and patient outcomes (Chien, 2019). The project aimed to translate evidence effectively into the project site by implementing the AHA, ACC, and TOS guidelines to achieve significant patient outcomes. The AHA, ACC, and TOS guidelines consisted of a one-page algorithm with evaluation and the corresponding interventions. This tool was the intervention implemented by APNs and was used as a visual aid to show the APNs and the patients the recommended interventions.

A Digital Scale and Health-O-Meter

The digital scale for measuring weight and health-o-meter professional wall-mounted height rod for measuring height were other data collection tools available at the project site. The digital scale was used to measure weight in pounds, and a health-o-meter was used to collect data on height, enabling the MA to calculate the BMI. To support the digital scale and health-o-meter tool's reliability, the participants were weighed on the same scale at the same project site to avoid scale-to-scale variability. The same MA used the same height measuring tool for all participating patients to support reliability. The self-reporting of height and weight by the participants was not accepted. Data were initially collected and recorded in the patient's paper chart by MA.

Validity

Validity is defined as the degree to which an instrument measures what it is intended to measure (Souza et al., 2017). According to Ryan et al. (2019), validity looked at the evidence used when interpreting the results. There are several validity types: face validity, content validity, criterion validity, and construct validity. The ORK-10 was an instrument created by Swift and colleagues to "validate a short, a reliable psychometric scale measuring knowledge regarding effects of obesity health" (Swift et al., 2006, p. 661). The ORK-10 had been evaluated for criterion validity by Swift et al. (2006). Swift et al. (2006) administered ORK-10 to individuals with no obesity-related expertise (n=230) and a sample of experts (n=200). Swift et al. (2006) hypothesized that participants with obesity-related specific knowledge would achieve significantly higher scores on the ORK-10 scale than participants with obesity-related no-specific knowledge, thereby establishing criterion validity. Univariate and multivariate statistical analyses were used to investigate the scale's criterion validity. The finding indicated that criterion validity was demonstrated by those with educational or vocational expertise in obesity who scored significantly higher than non-experts (median 9.0 vs. 4.0, Z= -17.364; *P*>0.001). The authors used Cronbach's alpha to assess the tool's validity, usually reported at 0.871. Therefore, ORK-10 had been deemed a valid tool for use in this project.

The AHRQ Tool 2 provided basic step-by-step instructions in conducting chart review. The toolkit was an evidence-based and reliable source that offered PCPs guidelines to properly manage overweight and obese patients (McGinnis et al., 2014). The AHRQ Tool 2 was reported as an evidence-based and valid source that offered step-by-step tools that providers could adapt to fit their clinical setting (McGinnis et al., 2014). To support the validity of AHRQ Tool 2, Melle et al. (2018) conducted a study to determine the validity and reliability of a medical record review using a chart audit scale for screening obesity. A convenience sample of 200 individuals aged 50 years and older were recruited from the outpatient clinics population. Validity was assessed using content, face, and construct validity. The Cronbach's alpha of the subscales ranged from 0.57 to 0.89 (Melle et al., 2018). The results suggest that the medical record review using chart audit form could be an appropriate measure for health record review related to screening for obesity.

The AHA/ACC/TOS guidelines, face and content validity were achieved through expect panels. First, the health professional validated the original instrument in managing overweight and obesity in primary care (Jensen et al., 2014). Then, as the instrument went through many revisions, content validity was established by high-quality randomized trials, meta-analyses, and observational studies by a panel of experts on each subject, including overweight and obesity (Jensen et al., 2014). The AHA, ACC, and TOS guidelines for the management of overweight and obesity in adults was adopted by several researchers used with a variety of ailments within various health agencies: The American Association of Cardiovascular and Pulmonary Rehabilitation, American Pharmacists Association, American Society for Nutrition, American Society for

Parenteral and Enteral Nutrition, American Society for Preventive Cardiology, American Society of Hypertension, Association of Black Cardiologists, National Lipid Association, Preventive Cardiovascular Nurses Association, The Endocrine Society, and National Coalition for Women with Heart Disease (Jensen et al., 2014). Therefore, AHA, ACC, and TOS referred to the guidelines as construct valid. The validity of the data collected using the digital scale and health-o-meter was supported by the primary investigator's actual measurements and not reported measurements from the participants. Validity was also supported by using devices to measure height and weight currently in the practice site. While the calibration date and time are unclear, the same device was used for the entire project; the overall outcome was to detect a weight change.

Reliability

Reliability is the extent to which a measuring procedure in quantitative research can be replicated and can provide the same result (Souza et al., 2017). It is an indicator that the instrument will maintain its performance regularly and produce similar results. Swift et al. (2006) used a cross-sectional survey to assess knowledge of obesity health risks (ORK-10). Questionnaires were administered to individuals with no obesity-related expertise (n=230) and a sample of experts (n=200). Swift et al. (2006) found criterion validity was demonstrated by those with educational or vocational expertise in obesity scored significantly higher than nonexperts (median 9.0 vs. 4.0, Z= -17.364; P>0.001). The Cronbach's alpha of the total scale was 0.83 in the researcher's study (Swift et al., 2006). Therefore, the ORK-10 demonstrated good internal consistency and established reliability. Swift et al. (2006) have stated that the ORK-10 can effectively evaluate a person's health information related to obesity risks. For this study, an acceptable score on the ORK-10 was 100%.

The AHRQ Tool 2 chart audit form was used to screen and track overweight and obese patients. The toolkit is an evidence-based and reliable source that offers crucial steps in providing tools that providers can adapt to fit their clinical setting (McGinnis et al., 2014). AHRQ Tool 2 was supported by AHRQ charged with supporting research designed to improve cost, address patient safety and medical errors. To support the reliability of this direct practice improvement project and the AHRQ Tool 2 chart audit form, Melle et al. (2018) conducted a study to determine the validity and reliability of a medical record review using a chart audit scale for screening obesity. A convenience sample of 200 individuals aged 50 years and older were recruited from the outpatient clinics population. Validity was assessed using content, face, and construct validity. A test-retest procedure was used to determine reliability by using Cronbach's alpha coefficient. The Cronbach's alpha of the subscales ranged from 0.57 to 0.89, and test-retest reliability ranged from 0.81 to 0.93, indicating a good range of reliability. The results suggest that the medical record review using chart audit form could be an appropriate measure for health record review related to screening for obesity.

Reis et al. 2018 conducted a qualitative study to determine participants' knowledge of obesity identification, evaluation, and management standards based on AHA, ACC, and TOS guidelines. A convenience sample of 200 individuals aged 50 years and older were recruited from the outpatient clinics population. Validity was assessed using content, face, and construct validity. A test-retest procedure was used to determine reliability by using Cronbach's alpha coefficient. The Cronbach's alpha of the subscales ranged from 0.57 to 0.89, and test-retest reliability ranged from 0.81 to 0.93, indicating a good range of reliability (Reis et al., 2018). The results suggest that the AHA/ACC/TOS guidelines could be an appropriate measure for assessing knowledge of obesity in an outpatient clinic.

The reliability of the digital scale and health-o-meter was determined by weighing participants on the same scale in the practice improvement project site to avoid scale variability due to variations in calibrations; the same height measuring device will be used for participants. Digital scales were used for the weight designed to weigh in pounds; a wall-mounted height measure was used to measure inches. All participants had their height measured with their shoes off and weight measured with their clothes; only data collected by the primary investigator using the specified measuring devices were used for reporting purposes.

Data Collection Procedures

Approval from the Grand Canyon University (GCU) Internal Review Board (IRB) was obtained before the initiation of the project (see Appendix A). After clearance from the project site and GCU, APNs and other staff were provided instruction on the project purpose and use of the AHA, ACC, and TOS guidelines for the project. Permission to use AHA/ACC/TOS guidelines was granted before implementing the project (see Appendix B). A copy of the AHA, ACC, and TOS guidelines was given to the APNs (see Appendix C). Due to the utilization of the ORK-10 questionnaire, Health Insurance Portability and Accountability Act (HIPPA) authorization forms were included and were signed by the participants. APNs also obtained consent forms before the intervention. APNs administered the ORK questionnaires pre-intervention and post-intervention on participants who were obese (BMI>30 kg/m2). The permission to use ORK-10 was granted for this project (see Appendix D). The ORK-10 questionnaire was used to determine obesity knowledge pre-intervention and post-intervention to determine if there was a change in obesity risk knowledge (see Appendix E).

The project manager began the paper charts audit after the project intervention phase. The patient paper charts were identified using chronological digit numbers starting with (1) as assigned during the intervention by APNs. Combined pre-intervention and post-intervention chart audits were evaluated to ensure participants met the inclusion criteria before the intervention. The inclusion criteria were adults with BMI greater than 25 kg/m^2, are between ages 18-64, have BMI less than 25 kg/m^2 reside in central California and be a patient at the primary project site. The exclusion criteria include a patient less than 18 or more than 64 years old. The patient paper charts were identified using chronological digit numbers starting with (1) as assigned during the intervention by APNs. A total of 28 charts were identified for review. The completed ORK-10 questionnaires were given to the project manager by the APNs at the end of implementing the AHA, ACC, and TOS guidelines. The project manager reviewed the pre-intervention and post-intervention ORK-10 questionnaires from 22 obese participants. The project manager did not have any direct contact, including telephone contact, with the participating patients throughout the project implementation.

The pre-intervention data (age, gender, medical history, height, weight, and BMI) and post-intervention data (weight and BMI) were collected from the patient's paper chart using AHRQ Tool 2 (see Appendix F). AHRQ Tool 2 provided step-by-step and detailed instructions for weight management tracking. For this project, weight management referral was not needed because APNs' adherence was not evaluated due to time constraints. Permission to use AHRQ Tool 2 was obtained (see Appendix G). All the data collected on the paper were secured in a folder and transferred to a Microsoft Excel spreadsheet kept on a separate flash drive specific to the data collected.

The flash drive was labeled and encrypted so that the project manager had only access to the drive. All the data collected from the patient's paper chart were secured in a locked drawer with a key at the project site available only to the project manager. Any printed data was shredded for confidentiality using the medical shredder available at the project site. No data was kept on a computer hard drive or viewed on unsecured internet access to maintain privacy and security of data at all times. Upon completion of the project, the collected data will be kept and preserved by the project manager for a maximum of three years and then be deleted.

Data Analysis Procedures

The clinical question guided the quantitative quasi-experimental project: To what degree did the implementation of Jensen's Guideline for the Management of Overweight and Obesity in Adults from the AHA, ACC, and TOS impact weight, BMI, and obesity risk knowledge when compared to current practice among adults with BMI greater than 25 kg/m^2 in a primary care clinic in central California? The data analysis aligned with the clinical questions and was appropriate for the research design. The data collected from the participating patient paper charts and ORK-10 score using a pencil and recorded into a Microsoft Excel spreadsheet. The specific raw data collected from participating patient paper charts were the age, gender, medical history, height, weight, and BMI on a sample size of 30 (n= 30) at the initial visit as pre-intervention and a sample size of 28 (n=28) post-intervention. The data was then entered into the SPSS 26.0 version. Patient outcomes of weight, BMI, and obesity risk knowledge were analyzed using a parametric paired samples *t*-test. The variables were then entered into frequencies, and all the frequency tables were run for each variable to check for missing values and incorrect data response category values (Knapp, 2018).

Descriptive statistics and a paired sample *t*-test were used to assess weight, BMI, and obesity risk knowledge for participating patients. A descriptive statistics and sample *t*-test were performed using SPSS version 26.0, and alpha was set to 0.05, indicating a *p*-value of less than 0.05 suggest statistical significance. In addition, a paired *t*-test was conducted to compare the mean value of weight loss, BMI, and obesity risk knowledge at pre-intervention and post-intervention and addressed the clinical question by evaluating the impact of implementing the guidelines on patient weight, BMI, and obesity risk knowledge. Nominal and ordinal variables from 30 participants were surveyed at baseline, and 28 participants post-intervention with frequency distributions.

Potential Bias and Mitigation

Certain limitations might have affected the outcome of the project. First, there may be chances of bias, mostly when the clinical question was answered using recorded data, leading to more errors and bias (McVay et al., 2018). This project provided an accurate representation of the impact of weight management in a primary care setting. Using a quasi-experimental design, significant bias to this project was the selection and sampling. The project used a sample of the final 28 participants from the project site's primary care setting, which posed selection bias. In addition, the participants were selected with inclusion and exclusion criteria from a single site to complete the survey, limiting the results' generalizability, which also posed a bias.

Ethical Considerations

The general codes in conducting human subject research are guided by the Belmont Report of 1978 (Adashi et al., 2018). According to the Belmont Reports, there are three fundamental ethical principles (respect, beneficence, and justice) regarding human subject studies. First, respect for individuals requires researchers to obtain informed approval from their research participants. The Belmont Report addresses informed consent as a necessary part of showing respect for all persons. It was now required that an individual involved in a human subject study understand what is being done in the studies (Adashi et al., 2018). Due to utilizing a questionnaire for this project, consent and HIPAA authorization forms required by GCU IRB were included. Participants were informed about the project procedure, the purposes, risks, anticipated benefits, voluntary participation, confidentiality, and anonymity. The participants were allowed to ask questions and that they have the right to withdraw from the project at any time. The primary investigator made sure that the participant's anonymity was maintained by giving the participants identification numbers. All documents were stored securely and can only be accessed by the primary investigator. Anonymity and confidentiality were maintained through the secure storage of private medical information and patient identity. The participants' and clinic's names were removed from all project materials and forms. The raw data will be stored for three years following completion of the study and then destroyed. Paper copies of data were shredded, and electronic files were encrypted for security purposes.

The beneficence means that all possible risks and benefits for participation must be clear to the participants. According to Adashi et al. (2018), the principle of Beneficence requires that potential benefits to the subjects are maximized, and potential risks of harm are minimized. The participants were about the benefits of the intervention. The project did not use any prescription weight loss medication or supplemental dietary products, posing minimal or no risk to the participants.

Justice means all participants should be treated equally. The selection of project subjects should be scrutinized so that no one is systematically selected based on race, ethnicity, class, or other factors (Adashi et al., 2018). The participants were chosen for reasons directly related to the project problem without considering any economic, social, and gender class. Compounding evidence of human suffering led the United States federal government to create the Institutional Review Board (IRB) process. This board regulates every aspect of research to ensure ethical considerations and the protection of human subjects.

This project followed all the procedures and protocols under IRB to ensure that this project would be conducted ethically with respect and protection for participants. (Adashi et al., 2018). There were no vulnerable populations involved in the project. Informed consent was available for those volunteering to participate; results were available upon completing the data collection and data analysis. The project results would be presented for dissemination to the DPI project committee, and a copy would be given to members of the project site personnel concerned with quality improvement. No conflict of interest was identified, and there was no involvement in the treatment regimen.

Limitations

The first limitation inherent in the project was the small sample size. The sample size can affect judgments of clinical significance (Tipton et al., 2017). A sample size that is too small reduces the power of the study and increases the margin of error, which can render the study meaningless (Tipton et al., 2017). The project used 28 participants, which resulted in the project not being generalized. A more diverse sample in the future regarding race and study location could help provide more insight about gaps for addressing overweight and obesity in adults in the primary care setting.

Another limitation was the project duration (four weeks), which was insufficient to evaluate the intervention's effectiveness for weight loss maintenance. According to Jensen et al. (2014), significant weight loss maintenance was achieved after three months of intervention. Weight management interventions were complex, mostly when the individual was not motivated or ready for a change. Therefore, drop-out was another limitation of this project. Bias was a potential limitation to this direct practice improvement project, especially as the sample did not accurately represent the overall population (Tipton et al., 2017). The participants were the patients who were known by the project manager and APNs from the project site. It was recognized that this project's positive outcome offered a chance for current practice to manage overweight and obesity in the primary care setting.

Summary

This direct practice improvement project was implemented to determine the effectiveness of the evidence-based AHA, ACC, and TOS guidelines on weight BMI and obesity risk knowledge in the primary care setting located in central California. The project used a quantitative method with a quasi-experimental design to determine if AHA, ACC, and TOS guidelines improved weight and BMI reduction and increased obesity risk knowledge. Overweight and obesity are serious conditions that required routine management, similar to other chronic diseases. A panel of experts from AHA, ACC, and TOS, among other stakeholders, developed a set of guidelines and recommendations for primary PCPs to manage overweight and obesity in adults (Jensen et al., 2014). However, the guidelines were not utilized as recommended (Jensen et al., 2014). The AHA, ACC, and TOS guidelines were introduced to treat overweight and obese adults at the project site.

The method of the project was quantitative descriptive statistics with a paired *t*-test. Data was collected using a pre-intervention and post-intervention chart audit. The data collected were the patient outcomes of weight, BMI, and obesity risk knowledge. The sample size of 27 participants was determined using a G* power analysis. The data was collected from 28 participants pre-intervention and post-intervention chart audits and handled appropriately and ethically in accordance with HIPAA and the Belmont Report of 1979. The clinical question was confirmed with the data analysis. The design was quasi-experimental to compare the participant's pre-intervention and post-intervention data.

This chapter discussed the project strategy plan through which the project was conducted, including a methodology, project design, population and sample selection, and instrumentation. The discussion of validity, reliability, data collection, and data analysis procedures were included in Chapter 3. One of the key subheadings of the chapter is the ethical considerations and limitations. The discussion illustrated the

Institutional Review Board's creation, a board that is now essential to human research regulations.

Chapter 4 will analyze the overall data analysis of the project as discussed in tables and figures. Descriptive data, including a narrative summary of the participants in the project, will be addressed. Data collection and analysis procedures will also be discussed in the chapter. Finally, the results of the project, including each outcome-specific outcome, will be addressed.

Chapter 4: Data Analysis and Results

The purpose of this quantitative quasi-experimental quality improvement project was to determine if the implementation of the American Heart Association, American College of Cardiology, and The Obesity Society (AHA/ACC/TOS) *Guidelines for the Management of Overweight and Obesity in Adults* would impact weight, body mass index (BMI), and obesity risk knowledge among adults with BMI greater than 25 kg/m^2. The project was completed over four weeks in a primary care clinic in central California. The quantitative direct practice improvement project was for APNs to utilize the AHA, ACC, and TOS guidelines on every patient who met the inclusion criteria, aiming to improve weight, BMI, and obesity risk knowledge. The clinical question examined in this project was: To what degree did the implementation of Jensen's Guideline for the Management of Overweight and Obesity in Adults from the AHA, ACC, and TOS impact weight, BMI, and obesity risk knowledge when compared to current practice among adults with BMI greater than 25 kg/m^2 in a primary care clinic in central California? The problem identified at the primary project site was that it was not known if or to what degree the implementation of the American Heart Association, American College of Cardiology, and The Obesity Society (AHA/ACC/TOS) *Guidelines for the Management of Overweight and Obesity in Adults* would impact weight, body mass index (BMI), and obesity risk knowledge among adults with BMI greater than 25 kg/m2. Relative to the problem identified, the problem statement reiterates the lack of evidence-based clinical guidelines for APNs to treat overweight and obese adults at the project site. Overweight and obese patients often were addressed during the office visits at the project site;

however, they were given little ongoing weight management guidance. The patients usually were told to watch their diet regardless of their class of BMI.

Chapter 4 discussed the descriptive data, including a demographic summary of the project participants. Chapter 4 also showed how the data were analyzed statistically using a paired sample *t*-test. The results of the data collected from the chart audit were presented and explained in this chapter. The specific outcomes, including the weight, BMI, and obesity risk knowledge, were presented. The chapter also showed how the data was analyzed statistically using figures and tables.

Descriptive Data

The project site was a primary care setting located in central California. This project's population was all adult patients, male and female age 18 to 64 with BMI > 25 kg/m^2 who receive care at the primary project site. The project sample included 28 participants, female (n=16) and male (n=12) completed the pre-intervention and post-intervention follow-up data collection. Table 1 provides the descriptive statistic data to describe the participants of the project. The mean age of the female and male participants was 38.96 years, with a minimum and maximum age of 22 and 62, respectively.

Table 1

Participant Demographics (N=28)

Variable	*M*	*SD*
Age	38.96	11.15
Gender	*n*	%
Female	16	57.1
Male	12	42.9

Table 2 displays the diagnoses of the participants. The most common medical diagnoses were hypertension (HTN), (n = 11, 39.3%) and hyperlipidemia (HPL) (n = 10, 35.7%). Seven patients (25%) did not have any medical diagnosis.

Table 2

Medical Diagnoses (N= 28)

Variable	*n*	%
Medical Diagnoses		
Asthma	1	3.6
Sleep Apnea	1	3.6
Hypertension	11	39.3
Hyperlipidemia	10	35.7
Chronic Low Back Pain	1	3.6
Chronic Back Pain	2	7.1
Type 2 Diabetes Mellitus	4	14.3
Depression	5	17.9
Pre-Diabetes	2	7.1
Substance Use Disorder	1	3.6
None	7	25.0

Data Analysis Procedures

The clinical question for this project was: To what degree did the implementation of Jensen's Guideline for the Management of Overweight and Obesity in Adults from the AHA, ACC, and TOS impact weight, BMI, and obesity risk knowledge when compared to current practice among adults with BMI greater than 25 kg/m^2 in a primary care clinic in central California? Patient outcomes of weight in pounds, BMI, and obesity risk knowledge were analyzed using a parametric paired samples *t*-test. The data values were matched, which indicated that the paired *t*-test would be the most appropriate analysis (Tipton et al., 2017). Therefore, a paired *t*-test was conducted to compare the mean value of weight loss, BMI, and obesity risk knowledge at pre-intervention and post-intervention to address the clinical question by evaluating the impact of implementing the AHA,

ACC, and TOS guidelines on patient weight BMI and obesity risk knowledge. Statistical analysis was conducted using SPSS version 26, and alpha was set to 0.05, indicating a *p*-value of less than 0.05 suggests statistical significance.

Results

The clinical question for this project was: To what degree did the implementation of Jensen's Guideline for the Management of Overweight and Obesity in Adults from the AHA, ACC, and TOS impact weight, BMI, and obesity risk knowledge when compared to current practice among adults with BMI greater than 25 kg/m^2 in a primary care clinic in central California? Three patient outcomes were assessed pre and post-intervention, including weight, BMI, and obesity risk knowledge.

Patient weight

A paired *t*-test was conducted to examine patient weight (in pounds) before and after the implementation of AHA, ACC, and TOS guidelines. The results are presented in Table 3. As shown in Table 3, there was a statistically significant reduction in patient weight from pre-intervention (M=201.00, SD=40.33) to post-intervention (M=197.86, SD=39.31), $t(27)=4.01$, p=.000. The average weight loss was 3.14 pound

Table 3

Paired t-Test Results Comparing Patient Weight at Pre-and Post-Intervention (N =28)

Patient Outcome	Pre-Intervention		Post-Intervention		*t* (27)	*p*
	M	*SD*	*M*	*SD*		
Weight in Pounds	201.00	40.33	197.86	39.31	4.01	.000

Figure 1 displays the average weight at pre-intervention and post-intervention for the 28 participants in the study. The total average weight loss at pre-intervention was four pounds.

Figure 1

Average Patient Weight (Pounds) at Pre-and Post-Intervention (N = 28)

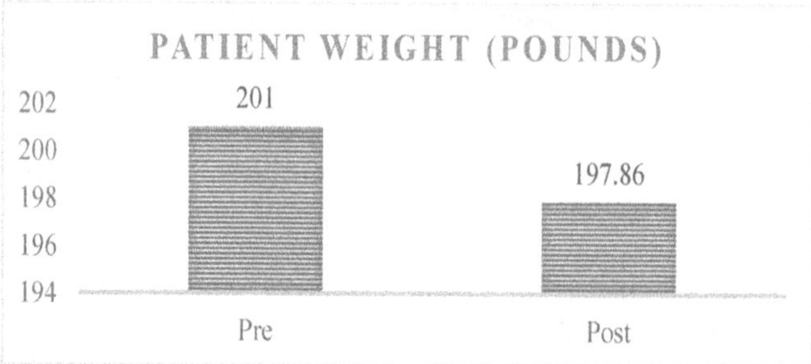

Patient BMI

A paired *t*-test was conducted to examine patient BMI before and after the implementation of AHA, ACC, and TOS guidelines. The results were presented in Table 3. As shown, there was a statistically significant reduction in patient BMI from pre-intervention (*M*=33.07, *SD*=6.25) to post-intervention (*M*=32.53, SD=6.11), *t*(27)=3.44, *p*=.002. The average BMI reduction was 0.83 points.

Table 4

Paired t-Test Results Comparing Patient BMI at Pre-Intervention and Post-Intervention (N = 28)

Patient Outcome	Pre-Intervention		Post-Intervention		*t(28)*	*p*
	M	*SD*	*M*	*SD*		
BMI	33.07	6.25	32.53	6.11	3.44	.002

Figure 2 displays the average BMI at pre-intervention and post-intervention on the 28 participants in the study. The average BMI decreased significantly from 33.07 at pre-intervention to 32.53 at post-intervention.

Figure 2

Average Patient BMI at Pre-Intervention and Post-Intervention (N = 28)

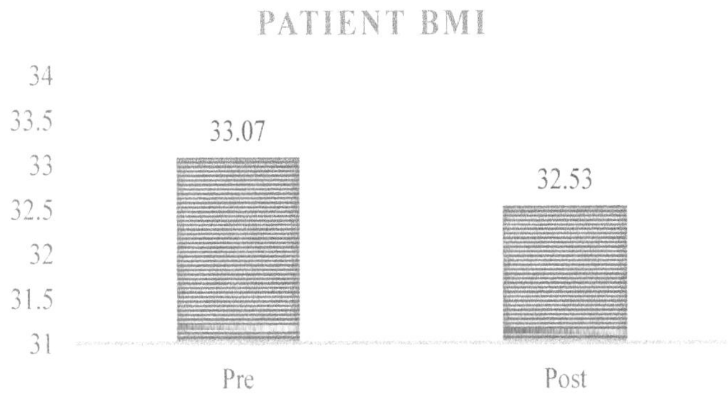

Obesity Risk Knowledge

The paired sample *t*-test showed a statistically significant improvement in obesity risk knowledge score from pre-intervention (*M*=5.68, *SD*=0.89) to post-intervention (*M*=9.50, *SD*=0.51), *t*(22)= -26.95, *p*=.000 (Table 4). The average improvement in obesity risk score was 3.82 points.

Table 5

Paired t-Test Results Comparing Patient ORK-10 Scores at Pre- and Post-Intervention (N =22)

Patient Outcome	Pre-Intervention		Post-Intervention		*t (21)*	*p*
	M	*SD*	*M*	*SD*		
ORK-10 Score	5.68	.89	9.50	.51	-26.95	.000

Figure 3 displays the average obesity risk knowledge score at pre-intervention and post-intervention for the 22 participants that completed the questionnaire. The average obesity risk knowledge score increased significantly from 5.68 at pre-intervention to 9.50 at post-intervention, on a scale from 0 to 10.

Figure 3

Average ORK-10 Score at Pre-Intervention and Post-intervention (N = 22)

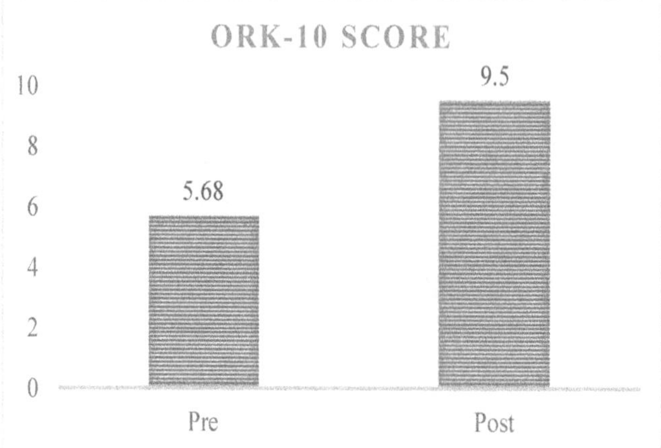

Summary

This quantitative-quasi-experimental direct practice improvement project used the clinical question: To what degree would the implementation of the American Heart Association, American College of Cardiology, and The Obesity Society (AHA/ACC/TOS) *Guidelines for the Management of Overweight and Obesity in Adults* would impact weight, body mass index (BMI), and obesity risk knowledge among adults with BMI greater than 25 kg/m^2 in a primary care clinic in central California? A total of 28 patients were included in the project. The patients' average age was 38.96, and most of the participants were female (*n*=16, 57.1%). Data for the patient outcomes of weight, BMI, and obesity risk knowledge were extracted from patients' paper charts. In addition, a paired *t*-test was conducted to examine average weight, BMI, and obesity risk knowledge before and after the implementation of AHA, ACC, and TOS guidelines.

The results revealed statistically significant improvement in patient weight from pre-intervention (*M*=201.00, *SD*=40.33) to post-intervention (*M*=197.86, *SD*=39.31), t(27) = 4.01, *p*=.000. There was also a statistically significant reduction in patient BMI from pre-intervention (*M*=33.-7, *SD*=6.25) to post-intervention (*M*=32.53, *SD*=6.11), *t*(27)=3.44, *p*=.002. Finally, the result showed a statistically significant improvement in obesity risk knowledge score from pre-intervention (*M*=5.68, *SD*=0.89) to post-intervention) *M*=9.50, *SD*=0.51), *t*(21)= -26.95, *p*=.000. This project demonstrated that the implementation of AHA/ACC/TOS guidelines had a statistically significant effect on patient outcomes. The results also supported meaningful clinical use, as all patient outcomes improved after implementing the AHA/ACC/TOS guidelines.

Chapter 5 compiled this direct practice improvement project in its completeness. The importance of the AHA, ACC, and TOS guidelines implementation and use were reiterated in the final chapter. A summary of the overall project and the findings and conclusions are discussed. The theoretical, practical, and future implications are also presented in detail. Lastly, the project manager offered recommendations for future projects and for future practice.

Chapter 5: Summary, Conclusions, and Recommendations

Adult overweight and obesity issues continued to rise despite the availability of published evidence-based clinical guidelines to help patients manage these conditions. The project sought to answer the clinical question: To what degree would the implementation of the American Heart Association, American College of Cardiology, and The Obesity Society (AHA/ACC/TOS) *Guidelines for the Management of Overweight and Obesity in Adults* would impact weight, body mass index (BMI), and obesity risk knowledge among adults with BMI greater than 25 kg/m^2 in a primary care clinic in central California? The independent variable for this project was the AHA, ACC, and TOS guidelines. The dependent variable was the patient outcomes of change in weight, BMI, and obesity risk knowledge. A quantitative research methodology was used for the project due to its ability to provide numerical data regarding the relationship between variables.

Chapter 5 will principally compile this quality improvement project in its entirety. After implementing AHA, ACC, and TOS guidelines, the intervention outcomes were reiterated in Chapter 5. Discussion of how the quality improvement project will contribute to future practice and project were discussed. Theoretical data analysis relative to the clinical question will also be addressed. Chapter 5 will conclude with both recommendations for future projects and recommendations for future practice

Summary of the Project

Overweight and obese patients were not identified or managed by APNs due to a lack of standardized clinical guidelines at the project site. A lack of established guidelines for overweight and obesity management at the project site led to a lack of intervention with patients experiencing overweight and obesity. Evidence-based clinical guidelines for managing overweight and obesity were not available at the project site. The project answered the clinical question: To what degree would the implementation of the American Heart Association, American College of Cardiology, and The Obesity Society (AHA/ACC/TOS) *Guidelines for the Management of Overweight and Obesity in Adults* would impact weight, body mass index (BMI), and obesity risk knowledge among adults with BMI greater than 25 kg/m^2 in a primary care clinic in central California? The project aimed to provide evidence-based AHA/ACC/TOS guidelines to APNs as a reference for treating overweight and obesity at the project site. This project demonstrated that the implementation of AHA, ACC, and TOS guidelines had a statistically significant effect on patient outcomes. The results also supported meaningful clinical use, as all patient outcomes improved after implementing the AHA, ACC, and TOS guidelines.

The patients usually were told to watch their diet regardless of their class of BMI. It was not known if or to what degree the implementation of AHA, ACC, and TOS guidelines would impact weight, BMI, and obesity risk knowledge compared to current practice among adults with BMI greater than 25 kg/m2. The project implemented a quantitative method for data collection and evaluated the effects on the dependent variables, weight loss outcomes (change in weight and BMI and increased obesity-risk knowledge). The independent variables, the AHA, ACC, and TOS guidelines, were measured using the AHRQ Tool 2 and ORK-10 questionnaire pre-intervention and post-intervention. The dependent variables were patient outcomes of weight, BMI, and obesity risk knowledge. The weight and BMI were measured with the same scale by the same MA pre-intervention and post-intervention. There was a clinically statistically significant difference in weight, BMI, and obesity risk knowledge from pre-intervention to post-intervention, supporting the clinical question.

Summary of Findings and Conclusion

This project site sought an evidence-based solution to address obesity and overweight in the primary. A quantitative, quasi-experimental design project with pre and post-intervention chart review with patients with BMI >25 kg/m^2 in a primary project site located in central California was evaluated. This project aimed to answer the clinical question: To what degree would the implementation of the American Heart Association, American College of Cardiology, and The Obesity Society (AHA/ACC/TOS) *Guidelines for the Management of Overweight and Obesity in Adults* would impact weight, body mass index (BMI), and obesity risk knowledge among adults with BMI greater than 25 kg/m^2 in a primary care clinic in central California? The results showed that the selected sample of 28 overweight and obese participants revealed statistically significant improvement in patient weight from pre-intervention (M=201.00, SD=40.33) to post-intervention (M=197.86, SD=39.31), t(27) = 4.01, p=.000.

The percentage of body weight loss by BMI categories was noticeably more significant among those classified as obesity class II with 1.90% (SD±4.34) followed by obesity class I with 1.59% (SD±4.07) and overweight 1.11% (SD±3.22). According to the AHA, ACC, and TOS guidelines, almost half of the participants selected showed positive weight changes. Among 28 participants who received intervention by APNs based on AHA, and ACC and TOS guidelines showed a significant difference between pre-intervention and post-intervention BMI. One of the significant findings from this project was the change in BMI, which showed a change of 3.44 points between pre-intervention and post-intervention. The project data concluded that implementing AHA, ACC, and TOS guidelines produced a statistically significant reduction in patient BMI from pre-intervention (M=33.-7, SD=6.25) to post-intervention (M=32.53, SD=6.11), t(27)=3.44, p=.002. Hall & Guo, 2017 counseled participants to follow a low-calorie of their choice, keep a food diary, and increase their physical activity to 150-200 minutes a week for 12 weeks. The finding indicated that individuals' dietary counseling included eating a low-calorie diet of their choice and increased activity level in weight loss programs.

The ORK-10 questionnaire was administered to the 22 participants with a BMI of 30 kg/m^2 or greater at pre-intervention and post-intervention to determine whether there was an improvement in obesity risk knowledge. The result indicated that the obesity risk knowledge score improved from 5.68 points (pre-intervention) to 9.50 points (post-intervention), indicating a statistically significant improvement in obesity risk knowledge score from pre-intervention (M=5.68, SD=0.89) to post-intervention) M=9.50, SD=0.51), t(21)= -26.95, p=.000 among obese patients.

Among the 22 obese participants, the four common medical diagnoses from this project were hypertension (n = 11, 39.3). This direct practice improvement project advanced scientific knowledge by challenging implementing overweight and obesity management in a primary care setting. Applying the AHA, ACC, and TOS guidelines confirmed that this type of intervention offered an efficient method to manage overweight and obesity in a primary care setting. The AHA, ACC, and TOS guidelines recommended a low-calorie diet of the patient's choice and walking 150 minutes per week to reduce weight and BMI. The four-week intervention demonstrated positive results in reducing weight, BMI, and increase in obesity risk knowledge. This direct practice improvement project showed positive results in improving overweight and obesity management at the project site when considering that this project was implemented for four weeks. One can assume that a longer duration can improve more weight loss and maintenance. The APNs at the primary project site played an important role in implementing the AHA, ACC, and TOS guidelines.

Implications

This project suggested a gap in practice that could be closed with a weight management program in the primary care setting by implementing AHA, ACC, and TOS guidelines. This practice gap could be completed by APNs offering evidence-based guidelines and encouraging the patient to walk for at least 150 minutes per week and eat low-calorie meals. Based on the literature review for this practice improvement project, one of the essential interventions that PCPs can offer their overweight and obese patients is counseling and encouraging a combination of exercises and a healthy diet recommended by AHA, ACC, and TOS guidelines.

Based on the project results, implications include considering AHA, ACC, and TOS guidelines at the primary project site. Project results clearly showed that implementing AHA, ACC, and TOS guidelines helped patients reduce weight and BMI and increase obesity risk knowledge. This direct practice improvement project's strength was that it revealed that implementing the evidence-based AHA, ACC, and TOS guidelines focusing on a low-calorie diet and physical (walking 150 minutes or more per week) and obesity risk had a significant impact on weight loss and obesity risk knowledge over four weeks.

Theoretical Implications

The results found in this project have the potential for theoretical implications suggesting the allowance of the implementation of AHA, ACC, and TOS guidelines by APNs at the project site to use the guidelines to recognize and treat overweight and obesity. One strength of this project was the positive result of answering the clinical questions. In addition, this project established the benefit of the AHA, ACC, and TOS guidelines utilized at the project site for managing overweight and obese patients. One of the project's weaknesses was that overweight and obese patients might not want to follow the recommended intervention leading to withdrawal from the program. By introducing the AHA, ACC, and TOS guidelines to APNs at the project site, overweight and obese patients presented for routine care visits would be assessed for obesity-related diseases and managed appropriately based on the guidelines.

The theory of goal attainment relied on the relationship between patients and their healthcare professionals (King, 1997). For this project, overweight and obese patients relied on APNs to achieve specific goals and objectives during overweight and obesity management. The chart audit review form was used to investigate the patient outcomes of weight and BMI. The relationship was manifested as a series of transactions in a primary care visit for managing overweight and obesity. If the APN was to address overweight and obesity, planning for implementing the nursing process must occur. This project set the foundation by leading the APNs to the point of readiness to implement and manage overweight and obesity using the AHA, ACC, and TOS guidelines in a primary care setting. The utilization of lifestyle modification in TGA application to manage self-image problems due to overweight and obesity has been a standard therapeutic strategy.

Lifestyle modification is recommended as one of the first approaches to obesity treatment. However, unsuccessful intervention can be a referral to obesity management for pharmacological or surgical interventions used in conjunction with lifestyle modification may be necessary.

This quantitative improvement project applied the TGA in identifying priority problems that require using interventions as established in AHA, ACC, and TOS guidelines. This theory proved to be helpful as the goals were formulated and set mutually by the overweight/obese patients and the APNs. The application of TGA highlighted the importance of overweight and obese patients' participation in decision-making and the process of nurse-client interaction that influenced the effectiveness of intervention for the attainment of goals. The AHA, ACC, and TOS guidelines as interventions were instrumental in assisting overweight and obese patients in increasing their level of adaptive response by developing a positive self-perception, enhancing interpersonal relationships, and improving social behavior when engaged in weight management programs. Consequently, attaining a positive goal for weight-loss management is evidenced by weight reduction from 201 to 197 pounds after the implementation period of four weeks. Based on the findings of this project, it is therefore concluded that the utilization of TGA
can serve its purpose to increase the level of adaptive response to reduce the weight of the overweight and obese patient by utilizing AHA, ACC, and TOS guidelines

The HBM focused on taking preventive measures to prevent or control the disease, such as overweight and obesity-related risks. The HBM represented the six concepts: Perceived susceptibility, perceived severity, perceived benefits, perceived barriers, cue to action, and self-efficacy (Rosenstock, I. M. (1974). According to a study by Saghafi-Asl et al. (2020), the application of HBM increased the participants' knowledge of obesity risk knowledge, dietary, and physical activity. Applying this theory to this project, obese individuals will be more likely to engage in lifestyle modification behaviors to manage their weight if they understand the seriousness and potential consequences of the obesity, understand their risk for developing the obesity-related disease, understand that following the recommended behavior change will reduce the risk or severity of obesity, understand the difficulties and cost of adopting behaviors, the internal or external motivations promoting the desired behavior, and understand their capabilities to perform a new health behavior successfully. The participating overweight and obese patients understood the relationship between caloric intake, activity, and exercise. They embraced health beliefs consistent with effective lifestyle modification outlined in the AHA, ACC, and TOS guidelines. Using the HBM, overweight and obese individuals identified their goals, actions steps, barriers, and commitment level to each goal

The project results show that understanding the risk of obesity-associated had a significant impact on weight loss outcomes. Integrating the HBM in the primary care setting for weight management could help APNs anticipate and describe health behaviors among overweight and obese patients. Patients who received intervention on obesity management with APNs were more motivated to follow intervention to prevent obesity-related diseases. The application of HBM on weight management behaviors could foster change to a healthy lifestyle. Applying these two theories to weight strategies helped overweight and obese patients engage in a low-calorie diet and physical activity behaviors to manage their weight if they know self-management and obesity risks. The AHA, ACC, and TOS guidelines, when combined with the HBM and TGA, showed success in gradually increase PA and low-calorie food through the four-week intervention, which led to an increase in weight loss. The HBM and TGA hold promise for guiding the design of intervention protocols for the future project into primary care weight management.

Practical Implications

The APNs were strategic facilitators of delivering best care practices for addressing adult overweight and obesity in the primary care setting. Although there were many evidence-based guidelines for managing overweight and obesity in a primary care setting, a lack of utilization of the evidence to meet adults' needs with overweight and obesity still exists. Implementing a quality improvement project utilizing the evidence-based AHA, ACC, and TOS guidelines provided an effective strategy to guide APNs in managing overweight and obesity at the project site. This direct practice improvement project was the first step in making positive changes in addressing the reversible condition of obesity. However, more projects were needed to assess APNs' knowledge of obesity risks and behaviors in utilizing recommended guidelines in their practice settings.

Future Implications

The future project's implication includes assessing the APN's understanding of obesity risks and impacts on overweight and obesity. Another implication is to examine if the treatment of obesity is closely aligned with the management of other chronic illnesses at the project site. Finally, another important implication for a future project is to examine the impact of collaborative practice agreements and the limitations they imposed on APNs, focusing on obesity rates and treatment rates.

This direct practice improvement project showed that weight loss outcomes were significant compared to post-intervention. This project's results revealed that implementing the evidence-based AHA, ACC, and TOS guidelines for weight management in the primary care setting could impact patients' outcomes of weight, BMI, and obesity risk knowledge. However, it was not known if the effects of this project, when implemented in other primary care settings or larger sample sizes, would provide the same result. APNs and other PCPs in the primary care setting could benefit from the development of this project.

Recommendations

This direct practice improvement project showed that implementing evidence-based ACA, ACC, and TOS guidelines in primary care settings significantly decreased weight, BMI, and increased obesity risk among overweight and obese patients. This project was an initial step in managing overweight and obesity in the primary care setting. APNs were experts in managing other diseases in a primary care setting. Therefore, they were equipped to address and manage overweight and obese patients using the established evidence-based AHA, ACC, and TOS published for PCPs. In addition, giving the APNs the AHA, ACC, and TOS guidelines would continue to identify and manage overweight and obesity at the project site.

Recommendations for Future Projects

This quantitative direct practice improvement project focused on overweight and obesity management and preventing obesity risks through evidence-based guidelines. The practice improvement project took place at the project manager's workplace with 28 participants and may not accurately represent all the primary care settings. The same results may not be elicited if the author or participants had to travel to the intervention and data collection location. Therefore, this similar project needs to be implemented at different primary care locations with higher volumes of participants.

Reviewing the results of the AHA, ACC, and TOS guidelines implementation at four weeks, three months, and six months in a primary care setting would be a conceivable future project using a quantitative method to determine if a similar result will be achieved. The project manager cannot say that the statistically significant findings in the four-week intervention will be maintained for a more extended period and may not also represent ongoing weight loss sustainability. It is unknown how long the participants would maintain weight loss. The current project was only four weeks of intervention, and long-term weight loss data would be needed to support findings because more significant weight loss outcomes are shown within three months of treatment (Bear et al., 2020).

Another recommendation for a future project is to use quantitative with pre-intervention and post-intervention to assess whether specific dietary or calorie recommendations by APNs would be beneficial for weight loss. A detailed nutritional or calorie prescription was not included in this project. It is important to know if more weight loss would be achieved when specific dietary or calorie was prescribed.

The intervention for this project included providing a low-calorie diet and physical activity counseling by encouraging participants to walk for at least 150 minutes per week. Medications and other interventions were also considered treatment (Bays et al., 2019; Garvey et al., 2016; Jensen et al., 2014); however, the pharmacotherapy interventions were not included in this project. Therefore, another recommendation for the future project is to use a quantitative method to examine the implementation of lifestyle modifications and pharmacological therapy to determine if more weight loss will be achieved.

Recommendations for Future Practice

Several requests can be made for further use in implementing this project. The first recommendation for future practice based on the project's results is implementing overweight and obesity management using the AHA, ACC, and TOS guidelines. The PCPs in a primary care setting should assess the weight and BMI of their patients, making sure that the appropriate recommendations are carried out based on AHA, ACC, and TOS guidelines.

Another recommendation for future practice is to implement weekly follow-up visits during the first four weeks and, after that, monthly for the next six months until the patient reaches weight loss. The project site did not have a specific time frame for follow-up for overweight or obesity management. The project data revealed that patients who were seen on the initial visit and follow-up in four weeks lost more weight. It would be recommended that participants schedule weekly appointments to increase participant accountability, promote retention throughout the intervention, and reinforce weight-related behavior change. According to Reis et al. (2018), weekly and monthly follow-up interventions were essential for patients with low weight loss outcomes and lack of motivation in weight management programs.

The final recommendation is to provide additional support using phone-based-guided intervention, especially during this Coronavirus pandemic. Lewis et al. (2019)

conducted a study that incorporated telephone support into the management of obesity. The addition of telephone support improved more weight loss outcomes when compared to face-to-face care alone (Lewis et al., 2019). Participants who received the addition of telephone intervention in the first four-month period lost 4.87 kg, compared with no weight loss (+ 0.38 kg) in the face-to-face only care (Lewis et al., 2019).

CPSIA information can be obtained
at www.ICGtesting.com
Printed in the USA
LVHW051642200423
744807LV00010B/447

9 787993 257949